Volume
1

NORTH SHORE PUBLISHING AND EDUCATIONAL SERVICES

Regina G. Chace, Ph.D.

The Best of Dr 911

Published by:
North Shore Publishing and Educational Services
Post Office Box 9865
Las Vegas Nevada 89191-0865
First Edition, 2002.
orders@dr911.com
http://www.Dr911.com

Unattributed quotations are by Regina G. Chace, Ph.D.

First printing 2002

Printed in the United States of America

Contents

Preface- Note To The Reader

Writing this book was far more challenging then I could ever have anticipated. Although I was prepared for the expected challenges such as "Writers Block," or delays due to production and publication, I could never have expected the devastating events that took place on the morning of September 11, 2001.

I was already fully engaged in the production of The Best of Dr911, collecting data and conducting research for an additional book I was preparing to write on the resilient emergency public safety professional and maintaining an active private practice and consulting firm following my resignation from the department when "9/11" occurred.

I will never forget how I felt sitting in my living room while I watched the second plane hit the world trade tower in New York City, and then when buildings collapsed upon themselves on streets I'd grown up walking, taking thousands of lives with them, I felt more helpless then I think I have ever felt in my entire life. My heart broke that day and I don't honestly know if it will ever heal completely from such a tremendous collective loss.

In the months that followed I found that I couldn't work on my book, or do my research. I could barely go to my practice. I felt lost. Nothing seemed to hold the same importance or value anymore. How could I work on something so "trivial" as a book when something so horrific had occurred? What was I thinking? Who would care about things like this anymore? Why should I? There were more important things to do, or were there? I had no answers for those questions that could satisfy me, and so I stopped, waiting for when something would begin to make sense again.

Like everyone, eventually I went on with my life. Like everyone, eventually I convinced myself that there was still meaning in things that I once remembered and held true. Like everyone, eventually my life seemed to return to "normal." I went back to writing. I finished this book. My novel came out. I went back to work, only this time back in uniform. But, the truth is that even to this day there are still moments when my heart aches so deeply I can barely stand it.

All those innocent lives lost in New York, at the Pentagon and in a field in Pennsylvania; all those brave people who gave of their lives that day to save the lives of others, and all those men and women who still have so much life left to live yet may one day soon give their lives in service to our country, we will never forget you.

Regina G. Chace, Ph.D., Las Vegas, Nevada

Acknowledgments

There are so many good and kind people who have contributed to the making of this book by their heartfelt willingness to share their lives, and their stories with me. To the men and women on the dispatch floor of the Los Angeles Police Department to the streets their courageous officers work on, from Sacramento PD, to San Diego, New York, Long Island, Texas and all across the country I thank you for making this book possible. You have taught me well and in ways I could never have expected. Your generosity, courage, strength, commitment of self and unfailing humor are a testament to the outstanding work you do every day. Thanks to your patience with me I've learned enough that I can finally pack away my asbestos pants. Special thanks go to my family, my sister Pat Salzman, my brother Arnold Chace, and to my friends and colleagues Donna Tracy, Dr Beverlee Longstreet, Colonel Barbara Hostetler, Major Laura Garner, Captain Tammy Tatreau, Detective Deborah Gonzales, Dr Azadeh Famili, and Dr Barbara Lepinski.

THE BEST OF DR 911.COM

The Suicidal Employee

Chapter 1

The Suicidal Employee

WHEN IT'S SOMEONE YOU KNOW...

Most supervisors and employees hope they never find themselves in the position of wondering whether a colleague, subordinate or coworker is at imminent risk for suicide. Disturbing at any time, completed suicides are particularly disturbing to those who are on the frontline and know first hand the traumatic impact of suicide on everyone involved, including the friends and family who are left behind. The effects are devastating, and no matter how hard someone tries to understand death by suicide it never really "makes sense." But suicide isn't about "making sense." It's about feelings and those feelings are not likely to make sense to anyone other than the person who is feeling them. As we know from research, suicide isn't so much about the desire for death as it is about the overwhelming need to end perceived pain.

Identifying The Risk

"This past year I responded to the suicide of a 22 year old male who was intoxicated and committed suicide with a shotgun to his head. 12 years earlier I had responded to a call at his mother's house when she reported him being sexually molested by his biological grandfather (her dad). Grandpa got a few years in the pen and was out. Recently the 22 year old had been living with Grandpa. He had never been the same since he and his sister were molested. The night before he committed suicide he and his girlfriend had been smoking marijuana and drinking heavily. He told his girlfriend what his grandfather had done to him and told her he was depressed. She went home about 2 am and tried to call him back at 4 am. His grandmother found him at 7 am when she tried to wake him for work.

At the time I worked the suicide I didn't put 2 and 2 together. I knew I was at Grandpa's house but didn't recognize who the kid was until the Medical Examiner was there. I thought, "I wish I could go over there and ask Grandpa how he felt when he killed his grandson at 12 years old." That's essentially what he did. It just took 10 years for him to finally die. But you can't do that, you just clear the call, do your paperwork and go on to the next thing."

When we are safely cloaked in our "professional gear," responding to a crime scene or dispatching on 911, we know what is expected of us. This is what we've been trained to do, and as one person said to me recently, "Trauma is my life, whether it's emotional or physical. I admit that I'm a masochist and I'm at my happiest when I'm dealing with other people's problems. Maybe it's my way of subconsciously ignoring my own, but it works."

Whether it's the first time or the fifteenth time our predetermined professional role serves to "separate" us from the reality of the traumatic event. In the professional literature this separation is called a "functional detachment or denial." Although we may not consciously realize we are doing this at the time functional detachment or compartmentalization of our feelings during a high stress incident enables us to function.

"At the time of the incident I didn't feel anything. My training took over and I did what I was supposed to do."

But what if the identified imminent risk isn't "out there" with John or Jane Q Public making suggestive life threatening statements? What if the warning signs we're reading are inside and much closer to home?

When these same warning signs are demonstrated by people we know and work with the decision to act can be far more challenging. We question our perception of what we hear or see and wonder whether intervention is necessary? What if we're wrong? What then?

When It's Someone You Know. For many of us working in emergency public safety, with already more than enough memories, thoughts, feelings and images left behind by completed suicides or traumatic deaths we've witnessed or responded to, the thought of a colleague, subordinate, friend or family member ending their lives in the same manner is extremely disturbing.

Even though we may know that anyone is vulnerable to depression and at-risk behavior, emotionally we struggle to accept this in someone we know and care about. Inadvertently, our own feelings and experiences concerning suicide interfere with our ability to perceive the seriousness of the situation.

In The Eye of The Storm

DR JANE

As an undergraduate student I worked part time as a research assistant in the university psychology department. One evening I received a phone call at home from a female graduate student who worked there with me. She was distraught over what she described as her failing grades. Although we'd never had a personal conversation before, outside of the University, I was flattered that she would call me, a younger student, to confide in. I was also understandably concerned when she disclosed how depressed she was.

We talked for over an hour during which time **she denied her suicidality** ("I would never do something like that"); **swore she had not disclosed her feelings to anyone else other then me** ("No one else would understand." and **thanked me repeatedly for helping** her ("I feel so much better. You've helped me more then anyone."), then **pleaded with me to keep her secret ("**You can't tell anyone! I would be so embarrassed if anyone knew.). I agreed. Approximately one month later this young student committed suicide.

As the students and faculty gathered on campus to share our grief we soon learned a startling fact. Inadvertently we had all participated in our young friend's demise. Each one of us present, senior as well as junior members of the department of psychology, students, Ph.D.s and M.D.s, in addition to two suicide hotlines and a variety of outpatient therapists, had all been contacted by this young woman at one time or another and each of us had been given the same information yet none of us knew about each other.

ONLY YOU

Each been told that he or she was the only person she had confided in. Each had been sworn to secrecy. Each had been thanked for being the "only one to help her" and each, out of concern for her and not wishing to jeopardize what they believed was her only outlet, (themselves) agreed to keep her confidence.

She was a colleague. She was a graduate student in psychology. She was an honors student. She worked as a research student in the Department of Psychology. People saw and spoke to her every day.

How had this happened? Her feelings made no sense to those whom she confided in and were obviously irrational but because each of us **prided** ourselves on our ability to understand human behavior, ("we were all in the field, after all,") and she "trusted" us with her confidence ("Only me.") we explained away her behavior. We denied the seriousness of her intent because it was so hard for us to accept that someone who lived and worked and studied in the very midst of a psychology department on a prestigious university campus could actually be suicidal without anyone noticing or taking it seriously.

We all told ourselves versions of the same story: that if she truly were at risk she would say so (she did) and that even if she didn't say anything, by some fluke of nature, then certainly one of the many, many mental health professionals she was surrounded by everyday would notice and intervene. **But no one did**.

The fact that she manipulated each of us by the information she selectively shared was little comfort. We contributed to the problem by allowing our personal feelings to get in the way. Call it arrogance, complacency and simple naiveté by choosing not to communicate with each other when the "Red Flags" were so clearly there we failed someone who was clearly in desperate need. *Our feelings interfered with our perceptions of the situation.*

The Emergency Public Safety (EPS) Professional.

As a psychologist I've spent many hours talking with public safety professionals who vehemently denied they would ever commit suicide or consider suicide an option "because I've seen what can happen to someone. I'd never do that to my family." Yet, months later these same individuals would make a suicide attempt after a crisis. *"I can't believe he killed himself. He seemed to be in such a good mood. He seemed happy."*

I've also spent equally as many if not more hours talking with public safety professionals who are so "high maintenance" and labor intensive in their needs that in a room of 20, he or she is the only person in the room one can focus on. The classic case of "20% of the people taking 80% of the resources." While these individuals are effective at alarming everyone in their presence with their provocative behavior and hundreds of potential "Red Flags," they never actually seem to follow through with what they threaten or imply. So, what do you believe and when is intervention appropriate?

Organizational Recommendations

The following sections represent some basic suggestions for your organization and for you professionally, as a supervisor, training officer or colleague. We will also cover you, as the human being, who may one day regrettably find yourself in positions you never wished for and hoped you'd never to go to.

Although not every possibility is listed, the following recommendations are those we feel any organization should consider as a baseline minimum for their employees. Modifications can be made according to the specific needs of the organization, based on size, location, personnel available, etc.

Supervisors often protect those personnel experiencing depression and deny the existence of any problems serious enough to warrant intervention by an outside source. However, such acts ultimately are a disservice to the affected personnel by denying them the help they need.

- **Personnel may resist seeking help.** Many fear that if help is sought, employment and economic security will be threatened. This myth can be dispelled through department policy and the approach utilized by responding supervisors.

- **Supervisors must be provided with adequate training and resources so that they**

themselves feel comfortable with approaching personnel who are potentially suicidal.

- **Education on depression and suicide should be implemented for all department personnel.** They should be informed that seeking help does not mean the end of their career, but the start of improving a new career. Asking for health signals strength and insight, not weakness and denial, and that must form the foundation of any prevention program.

- **A suicide prevention program can only work if members of the department feel free to take advantage of it.** Administrators and supervisors must play a nonpunitive role. They must be sensitive to the possibility that *any intervention provided may be experienced by personnel as stressful and threatening.* They must communicate to personnel that seeking help will not result in job termination, all information will be kept confidential, that other ways exist for dealing with a situation, no matter how hopeless it seems at the time and that someone is available to help them deal with their problems.

Training, policy and procedure must be set and communicated consistently across every level of department leadership by word and practice every day.

Integrity of thought and action are vital. If what you say isn't what you do, either individually or organizationally, then others will know this. Don't assume that because you're a "good player" no one will notice. They will. They may not say anything but they will notice that "what's good for the goose isn't what's good for the gander," and one of the most important factors necessary for making all this work will be missing: trust. Without it, all the policy and procedures in the world will do nothing to stem the tides of disharmony and poor morale. Your "word" and the word of your organization are really all you have. Once you allow that to lapse the road back is very hard to find.

When It's Someone You Know

Sometimes the red flags just keep on coming, and when it's someone you know taking the next step can feel like the longest mile you've ever traveled. While this is by no means an exhaustive list take time to review its contents. Consider the message embedded within: No one has a crystal ball, not even the professionals. Should personal factors come into play, simply be mindful of them, and repeat this key phrase to yourself:

"When in doubt, refer them out. Consult, consult, consult."

You must be abundantly clear and extremely honest with yourself when reviewing this list and looking within. The consequences of denial can be deadly.

List of 16

1. ☐ Is the person you're concerned about someone you know well? A friend on the job? A close working associate or colleague? A subordinate you've developed a good working relationship with or who may have at one time been your trainee or probationer?

2. ☐ Do you admire, respect or look up to this person? Do you see him or her as your role model, mentor, or perhaps even the consummate leader and professional? Was he or she instrumental in your professional development, or you in theirs?

3. ☐ With this same individual in mind, whether you are peer-to-peer, or subordinate to supervisor, does your professional relationship include on duty or off duty socializing and the exchanges of confidences?

4. ☐ Is this someone whom you ordinarily seek out after particularly difficult calls, runs, or critical incidents?

5. ☐ Whether you have ever confided this information to another living soul or not, if you are really honest with yourself at this moment in time, have you ever felt significantly depressed or despondent to the extent that suicide, or placing yourself in harms way in whatever fashion, has been or is a viable option for you? (Consider the feelings

with this one, and not the words you may have said.) Are you feeling this way now? If this is an experience from your past, do you currently harbor feelings of shame, remorse or guilt for that particular time in your life?

6. ☐ Despite the potential for adverse consequences, and maybe even because of it, do you place yourself in high-risk situations? (For example: respond to shots fired without wearing vest; high speed pursuit without being belted in; extreme sports to the detriment of other activities or self-care; multiple affairs while married or in committed relationship; repeated abuse of substances; first on scene without calling for backup.)

7. ☐ If you were the first on scene of a completed suicide, suicide/homicide, did you see the body? Were you debriefed? Was there follow-up?

8. ☐ Were the victim's family, children, significant other, parents or friends present, and if so were they extremely emotional? Did you interact with them directly?

9. ☐ Have you ever been or were you routinely tasked with the responsibility of providing death notification(s) on one or more occasions? Of someone you knew to people you know or still know?

10. ☐ Has someone known to you in your division or command committed suicide?

11. ☐ Has a parent, adult caretaker; significant other, child or close family member ever experienced chronic bouts of acute depression, and/or suicidal ideation? Was a suicidal attempt ever made? Did this occur when you were a child or as an adult, and if the answer is both, was it continuous or on more then one occasion? If a suicide attempt was made did you provide intervention? If a completed suicide occurred did you find the body? Was there support provided to you in the aftermath? Do you still think about this event now

12. ☐ As a child and then later as an adult, did you experience feelings of shame, embarrassment, humiliation, frustration or anger towards someone you were close to because of the circumstances created by his or her depression? Did you ever tell him or her, or anyone else, how you felt about the experience and your subsequent feelings? Were you honest? Were you honest with yourself? If you've never told anyone, why not?

13. ☐ Have you had one of more instances of providing first response or first point of contact to a protracted critical incident, such as a barricaded suspect suicidal, or barricaded suspect with hostages? Bombing? Plane crash? Public display of violence with fatalities (PDVF)? Were children involved?

14. ☐ Have you dispatched on one or more calls in which the caller completed the suicide while talking to you?

15. ☐ Did a successful rescue attempt by you ultimately result in negative consequences for one or more victims? (For example, the victims were saved but later succumbed to their injuries in the hospital. Their final days were painful for themselves and their families. You were witness to their pain and grief.) Was there media attention immediately following the rescue to the extent that your actions were highlighted, or portrayed as heroic?

16. ☐ Do you have a strong personal faith or practice a spiritual belief in which suicide is considered an act against God?

Note how many and which items you have endorsed on the List of 16 then refer to **Table 1** for additional guidelines. Also note that additional information pertaining to supervisors, partners, friends and family members directly follows this section.

Table 1.

Red Flags	Number of Items Endorsed	Action Plan
One Red Flag	One endorsed Item	**No impact to mild impact.** Proceed with a healthy awareness. Consultation optional but not mandatory. Referral out optional.
Two Red Flags	Two endorsed items	**Mild impact to moderate impact.** Your experiences warrant mild to moderate concern for consultation. You judgment may be impacted by your own experiences. Consider referring out.
Three Red Flags	Three endorsed items	**Moderate impact.** Your ability to remain unaffected by your past experiences unlikely to very unlikely. Consultation and referral out strongly recommended.
Four Red Flags	Four or more endorsed items	**Serious impact.** Your past experiences will impact your judgment and perceptions. Consultation and referral out mandatory. Strongly consider follow-up consultation.

RESULTS

If you've endorsed items **5, 6, 11, 12 or 13 with Plane Crash, Bombing or PDVF with Children** consider this an automatic Three to Four Red Flags.

The average emergency public safety professional is likely to endorse two or more Red Flags during the course of his or her career.

Consequently, when faced with numerous Red Flags flying around someone you know, and know well, you may not be able to see the forest for the trees. At no fault to you, your perception may be skewed, influenced or biased by your own thoughts, experiences and feelings related to your job. This does not mean that you are incapable of acting appropriately or providing a realistic assessment or following your organizations pre-determined protocol for managing such situations. However, getting to that next step may be the mitigating factor.

Given your acknowledgment of one or more of the above, then consider this:

There may be times, circumstances and situations when you may not be the best person for making the critical decision.

Your reaction or response to a despondent employee, professional friend or colleague may be disproportionate to the actual needs of the individual, or their safety and well being, and that of the responding agency. Despite, and perhaps even because of your own years of experience with handling people and circumstances like this as a public safety professional, you may not always see as clearly when it comes to someone you know. Your heart may be in the right place, but your mind may not. You may want to do the right thing, but your ordinarily clear vision may be obscured by your own feelings about suicide, and traumatic death as well as your feelings about the person involved.

This in itself does not have to be an obstacle to providing an appropriate response. However, maintaining a conscious awareness of where you are on the continuum of feelings and how and when they may influence your actions is vitally important.

Interviews with suicide survivors tell us the actual window of time during which they are at greatest risk for attempting suicide is extremely small. If appropriate intervention is provided quickly the impulse to suicide fades and may not resume again. Consequently your next step is an important one.

Best rule of thumb, when it comes to someone you know:

When in doubt, refer them out. Consult, consult, consult.

Don't be alone in making such an important decision. You may think that you are maintaining confidentiality or protecting someone you care about from unnecessary stress by not telling someone else, but the consequences of not acting can be fatal. You will also live for a very long time with the memory of your decision.

Consulting with someone else (a professional, a supervisor, a trusted friend and colleague) is particularly important if you've endorsed two or more on the list above, and the person in question is actively presenting with symptoms and behavior that are of serious concern to you. The closer you feel to that person, the harder it may be to decide what to do, but if the Red Flags are showing up on the horizon, trust your feelings. The Red Flags wouldn't be there if something wasn't going on. Better to err on the side of caution then to risk someone's life.

Anything you choose to do can be done carefully, and with kindness and respect.

The intention of your actions should reflect the care that you feel and the integrity of your beliefs. You are acting to preserve the person, and the relationship, not just to follow standard operating procedures. If you're genuine in your intent, most people you are close to, even those in crisis and those you don't know, will feel that and know it. They will try to meet you where you are. If you are not genuine, they will feel that and know that, too. If you are not the best person for the approach, and you may not be, (There's no shame to this.) "**When in doubt, refer them out. Consult, consult, consult.**" No matter how responsible you may feel for your friend and or colleague, you really are not the only person capable of helping. Let someone else try.

"You talk about raising the Red Flags and you list 16 things that can and should raise a Red Flag in an employee or coworker. Christ, I answered yes to most of them and I feel I am a well-adjusted person who just happens to deal with death on a regular basis.

Our agency regularly offers critical incident debriefings to any employees who have experienced or handled a critical incident. In homicide we have experienced awful human suffering almost daily but we all successfully practice "functional detachment and denial." We are too busy to think about the tragedy of an incident and there is always a new case that quickly replaces the current investigation. I don't know how we coped with what we do but we all seem to have developed that "thick skin" to shield ourselves. I suppose the reason is we don't know most of our victims even though we can relate to some of them.

I have been involved in the investigation of three employees who have committed suicide. In one of the cases I personally spoke by telephone to a deputy just minutes before he shot himself to death. My conversation with him threw up numerous Red Flags and I called for rescue and patrol deputies to respond to his residence immediately. He killed himself in the time it took responding units to arrive.

I believe that because of my experiences I do recognize the danger signs when others will often rationalize. Your motto, **"When in doubt, refer them out. Consult, consult, consult,"** is something we stress in our agency although I know we have employees who wouldn't recognize a clue if it hit them in the face."

If, after reading this chapter, you find you would like additional more detailed explanation of the List of 16, please go the section entitled, "**Oh Say Can You See, The Red Flags Flying Over Me**."

Guidelines For Understanding Suicidal Behavior

Although there are many lists and formats that are available to help you in this process, the following represents a list intended on providing guidelines for understanding suicidal behavior and coping with the aftermath. It is by no means all-inclusive and there may be other methods or aspects that are not covered in this material. This list can also serve as a stand-alone presentation or hand-out during roll call.

If you find information that is more relevant to you, your situation, or even your temperament and personality we encourage you to use it. In fact, we also encourage you to share this material with whomever you can wherever and whenever appropriate. There can never be too much good resource information on hand.

What Motivates Someone To Consider Suicide As A Viable Option?

- A Cry for Help – feeling helpless and hopeless

- As a manipulation or means of control, feeling helpless, out of control, trying to get a response from other people, attempting to regain perceived power

- To end physical and/or emotional pain and suffering, overwhelming feelings of sadness, depression, anxiety, despair

- Anger

- There appears no other alternative.

Indirect Methods or Signs of Suicidal Intent or Suicidal Ideation

- Excessive risk taking on the job – putting self in harm's way (not wear flak jacket, not calling for backup when needed, antagonizing an already volatile situation unnecessarily, reckless driving)

- Excessive risk taking elsewhere

- High risk behaviors – not perceiving or acknowledging danger where danger exists
- Drinking and drug abuse
- Non-compliance with prescribed treatment or medication
- Provoking confrontations with dangerous individuals
- Reckless driving and car accidents, falls and other "accidents"

Direct Methods

- Any lethal method

Possible Early Warning Signs

- Hopeless and helpless statements, "Things will never get better."
- Suicidal statements: overt and implied, "Maybe I should kill myself", "My life is over", "I'm on the edge", or "I'm losing it"
- Depression and/or excessive crying

- Recent loss coupled with a decline in functioning – "I can't go on because of / or without ________"

- Statement of worthlessness, self-hate, and intense guilt, "I was never any good at relationships anyway."

- Angry statements such as, "If I can't have him or her, then no one can."

- Statements that suggest over identifying with someone who committed suicide, "I wish it were me;" "If someone like him could do it then anyone can."

- Getting affairs in order – giving away personal possessions

- Any evidence of indirect or direct methods of suicidal behavior ("practicing," storing or "hording medications," suspicious signs of "cutting" on self or evidence of self-injurious behavior, etc.)

Possible Interventions With Someone Exhibiting Early Warning Signs

- **Offer to talk to and be with the person.** Listen and don't feel responsible for being "the problem solver." You don't have to "fix it." You just have to be mindfully genuinely present. Many times that in itself is a gift to the person who is hurting and can do wonders for mitigating the circumstances.

- **Ask the person if they are having thoughts of hurting themselves.** Many people are extremely anxious about asking this question, as though voicing their concerns will "push the other person over the edge." Again, as long you are genuine in your intention and respectful and caring in your approach, many times hearing the words out loud from outside of themselves is a tremendous relief to the troubled person.

- **Show concern without trying to take control.** Control might be something you are used to having given your professional role and responsibilities, but this is one situation where you do not "hold the ace in the hole."

- **Involve significant others.**

- **Refer the individual to a mental health professional or crisis intervention facility.**

- **Call 911.**

- **Involve the supervisor.** Tell someone if you have any doubts. It's better to be safe than sorry.

"WHEN IN DOUBT REFER THEM OUT

CONSULT, CONSULT, CONSULT"

Normal Reactions to Someone Exhibiting Suicidal Behavior or Intent

Different people have different reactions to the suicidal behavior and suicide of another person, depending on their relationship with that person and their own life circumstances. However, some normal reactions to this kind of event can be expected.

Emotional

- Concern, surprise, disbelief
- Numbness, detachment
- Overwhelmed, lost, vulnerable
- Feeling abandoned, alienated, disenchanted, disillusioned
- Generalized anxiety
- Identifying with the person
- Helplessness, feeling like a failure
- Fear, guilt
- Anger, wanting to blame, irritability
- Uncertainty of feelings, confusion
- Spaced out, lost

Cognitive

- Self-doubt, replaying old conversations and thinking, "I should have seen it coming", or "What did I miss?" or "If only I had..."
- Preoccupation with the person and the situation; can't stop thinking about them.
- Taking on the characteristics and concerns of the suicidal person; becoming over responsive or responsible for their feelings or behavior.

- Increased or decreased awareness of the surroundings.
- Heightened or lowered alertness.
- Preoccupation with vulnerability or death.
- Poor concentration, flashbacks, distressing dreams.
- Memory problems, calculation difficulties, losing things.
- Difficulties with decision-making.
- Spiritual crisis; a questioning of religious or spiritual beliefs.
- Confusion, lowered attention span.
- Suicidal ideation without action or intent.

Behavioral

- Change in activity level, withdrawal, or clingy behavior.
- Less or more communicative than usual.
- Change in interactions with others, excessive gallows or morbid humor.
- Increased or decreased food intake, increased smoking, increased spending.
- Overly vigilant to environment.
- Increased alcohol intake without awareness of consequences or with the intention of exacerbating circumstances.
- Avoidance behavior.
- Acting out, antisocial acts, angry outbursts
- Suspiciousness

Physical

- Nausea, upset stomach, diarrhea
- Muscle aches, feeling uncoordinated, shakes, tremors
- Fatigue, sleep disturbance
- Profuse sweating, chills, rapid heart rate
- Headaches, vision problems, dry mouth
- More frequent visits to the physician for nonspecific complaints

Grief and Bereavement Process Following A Completed Suicide or Serious Attempt With Injury

- Denial- "This can't be happening!"
- Anger- "How could something like this happen!"
- Bargaining- "If only...!"
- Depression- "This is sad."
- Acceptance- "Sometimes bad things happen to good people."
- Not everyone goes through all the stages in order, or according to a set time frame in which feelings will be resolved. Allow yourself, or others, the time needed to work through it. When you're ready to move on, you'll know.

Coping Strategies

1. **Talk about thoughts and feelings with people you trust and feel safe with.** In fact, we recommend that you talk "until you're blue in the face." In most cases, there is no such thing as talking too much.

2. **Connect with others.** Don't set yourself apart or convince yourself that this is something you have to do on your own. Don't suffer alone.

3. **Get rest but avoid boredom.** Maintaining a normal activity level with positive interests and distractions and resting when fatigued is instrumental to healing healthily.

4. **Eat well.** This means eat foods that will replenish your life and vitality and give you the energy you need to cope effective. Limit your intake of "empty calories", foods you know offer nothing beneficial to you beyond satisfying a need to eat or do something with your time and feelings. Limit caffeine, sugar, fat, salt.

5. **Drink more fluids** (water and fruit juices are best); eat complex carbohydrates, low-fat and nonfat foods.

6. **Avoid excessive alcohol or over dependence on over the counter substances.** If you are unable to sleep, or are experiencing excessive behavioral or physical symptoms beyond a reasonable amount of time see your family practitioner or alternative health care provider. Err on the side of caution. Emotional experiences can manifest in very real physical symptoms that may require professional evaluation and intervention.

7. **Should this event receive media attention, limit your direct exposure and the direct exposure of those involved to the most common forms of media**, such as television, cable, newspapers and radio, for at least the first few days.

   If you or any first responder member of your work unit are asked to report on the event through media interviews include someone from your organization, such as press and media relations, to act as support and run interference. **Unsupported or overexposure to the impact of a potentially relentless media, either directly or indirectly, can retraumatize the individual unnecessarily.** Use caution. If this cannot be avoided then make certain those involved receive follow-up support services.

8. **Engaging in physical exertion, and exercise as soon as possible after demobilization is extremely helpful.** However, keep in mind that the goal of working out is facilitating the body's normal process of elimination of potentially damaging stress chemicals. Keep the work out to a level of moderate intensity.

9. **Try to restore normality to your daily routine as soon as possible and, when you are ready.** Maintaining normal routines, no matter how small have a "grounding effect" on most people, and will help you reclaim a life you may feel has been shaken by the event. However, also give yourself permission to change things up a little when needed, such as letting go of task you might ordinarily do so as to spend time with a supportive friend or family member.

10. **Maintain working, if possible.** The daily structure and routine will help normalize the situation and provide a grounding element that may be needed and welcome.

11. **Allow yourself time to grieve and heal.** There's no time schedule.

12. **View your reactions as normal reactions to trauma.** Let yourself "off the hook." Being a professional in emergency public safety does not mean that you "should" not have feelings or that you should get over them sooner and more readily then someone else. . In fact, all to the contrary, it may mean that the successful resolution of your feelings and reaction may be more complex because of your experience and background. Give yourself the room to be human. It's not a bad thing. Honest.

13. **Allow yourself the freedom to talk about your reactions to what happened with non-judgmental listeners.** Choose carefully, however. A judgmental critical listener may reinforce your fear that it's not safe to express your true feelings. This is not a good thing and is counterintuitive to the healing you will need.

14. **Seek peer, clergy, or professional assistance as necessary.** While not everyone has experience with emergency public safety professionals, there are many wonderful, supportive and competent professionals who are more then willing and able to help you or our colleagues. Use them; that's what they are there for. If you have a spiritual practice, even if long gone and neglected, this is the time to resurrect it.

15. **Don't be afraid** or embarrassed to draw comfort from any resource or avenue potentially

available to you, no matter how many years it's been since you've been to church, confession, the temple or wherever.

16. **Work on accepting that anyone in your situation would have responded similarly.** When it comes to someone who is close to you, professional or personal, no one can be certain how he or she will respond to a critical event until the moment is upon us. Again give yourself room to be human. You are. Don't become another statistic.

17. **Be gentle with yourself.** Move away from beating yourself up. No one has a "crystal ball." No matter what you think you knew or didn't know, no one has the ability to predict someone else's behavior with 100% accuracy. If someone tells you they do, they're wrong. If you think you do, you're wrong. Give it up. Let this one go. Resistance is futile. Holding on to it is only finding a way to punish yourself further. You don't need it.

18. **Consider using this crisis as an opportunity for growth, healing and positive change.** Refocus your goals and energy on what is really important to you. Hug your kids. Love your friends and family members. Remember to be affectionate with your spouse or significant other. Be kind to yourself.

19. **Allow yourself to be cared for by others.** Let them get close enough to love you, or at least express caring feelings. Stoicism is not always the best defense. Sometimes the best defense is no defense. "The walls that keep you safe, also keep you isolated and lonely." This doesn't mean give an open door policy to everyone in your division, but if you're too busy defending yourself against potential intruders, you also sever any potential opportunities for support. Be discreet and selective. Try giving yourself the opportunity to be known by someone who truly cares for you. It can help.

20. **Attend and participate in a debriefing**. If none is offered by your department seek one out on your own. Remember to follow up with additional contacts if one session feels inadequate. You may have to ask for this or actively seek out services on your own. You may have to be persistent. Do it. You are worth it.

When to seek additional assistance or help:

- Persistent intense feelings of discomfort. Unusually intense family conflicts that are out of the ordinary for your family or relationships.
- Significant symptoms that persist longer than four to six weeks (emotional, behavioral, physical). Unable to use traditional methods for self-soothing.
- Persistent suicidal thoughts and/or suicidal planning.
- Feel as though you are losing control of your impulses or losing conscious awareness of your behaviors or actions.
- Other self-destructive acting-out that is atypical for you or intensified, (sexual, financial, aggressive, or substance).
- Extreme behavioral changes such as increased inhibition, social isolation, cutting off of most normal contacts, behaviors or friendships.
- Persistently checking in with yourself or others to see if you're "normal."

Where To Seek Assistance

- Licensed psychologist or other health care provider in your local area.

- Employee Assistance Program or Peer Counseling Program

- A peer who has been through a similar situation, and with whom you feel comfortable.

- A mental health worker or counselor through your health plan.

- Clergy member of your church, temple or other organized religion or spiritual faith.

Special Notes

Supervisors

Being a good supervisor can be a tough job on any day of the week, but it's particularly challenging when navigating the proper channels for managing certain types of emotionally laden situations such as suicide.

No one expects you to "have eyes in the back of your head," but should you know first hand that a subordinate has had a family member, child, spouse, friend, partner or loved one suicide in the past, taking a few extra minutes to check in with him or her when he or she is the first responder or first point of contact in a suicide can go a long way towards preserving the quality of life for someone and reducing the potential for stress related problems in the future.

This is particularly important if the suicide victim is a child or someone known to the individual, such as a partner or friend.

Many supervisors feel pressed for time in a schedule that is already significantly overextended. Given their daily pressure cooker of commitments many supervisors I've spoken to are reluctant to say anything at all, either because of their own anxiety or discomfort about the topic in general and their lack of available time, or privacy issues when it comes to someone they know. They don't want to say the wrong thing so they don't say anything at all. They assume that if this individual needed something from the division, or the supervisor, that he or she would say so.

First line of approach: Don't make assumptions.

Showing genuine concern for the well being of an employee or subordinate is worth its weight in gold. You don't have to write a speech or block out a massive chunk of time in your schedule. It can be as simple as saying a few words, "I heard you were the first responder on the suicide of that 13 year old last night. I just wanted to check in with you to see how you're doing," and wait to hear and listen to the answer.

You don't have to fix anything. You don't even have to comment on what they say, just listen and then wish them well, let them know you're available and go on with your day. Most people are not going to tell you the "whole story," their life's history and then how they felt when they rolled out to the crime scene last night, but they will appreciate your awareness of the potential impact it might have on them and they will remember this.

If you show someone genuine concern you communicate by your actions and behavior that you value that person as a human being. This will go a long way towards maintaining the morale of that person, and of your division.

A 13 Year Old Boy Named Jack

One of the most significant calls I ever rolled out on was the suicide by hanging of a 13 year old boy. His mother had died the year before. That evening he had dinner with his father, brother and friend, played a game of Nintendo, and then went up to his bedroom. Minutes later his friend found him in his father's bedroom. He had taken several of his father's neckties and hung himself from a hook on the closet door. The family called 911 and both emergency medical and police were dispatched on the call. The responding officers were in the neighborhood at the time the call was broadcast and arrived within minutes. The boy was still alive. The responding officers joined in with the paramedics to assist in saving this young boys life. Unfortunately they were unsuccessful and he coded on scene.

I was called out to respond to the division and I was there when the 4 officers returned from the hospital.

You may wonder if requesting that a psychologist respond to a division following a suicide is standard operating procedure. It is not. In a city as large as Los Angeles if I had to respond every time patrol responded to a suicide, sadly, I might as well live at the division. There are far too many for this type of direct response, but there were several factors about this call that made it a particularly significant one.

First significant factor: the age of the victim. As I heard repeatedly that night, from each officer, "What does a 13 year old have going on in his life that's so bad that he kills himself? I didn't think about things like suicide when I was 13! How could a kid this young feel so hopeless?"

Second significant factor, four out of four officers had young children in their lives and in their homes, (sons and daughters, nieces and nephews). All four officers were experienced tenured officers and yet this suicide rocked them back in their seats. They openly cried during their individual debriefings as they talked about their feelings. Why? Because when they arrived on scene the boy was still alive and as they worked with paramedics to keep him alive they were reminded of the children they had at home. They saw their own sons and daughters in the face of this young boy, and they witnessed their own anguish and grief in the eyes of his father. The boy's suicide was so unexpected, and ultimately unpreventable. The officers were reminded that no one is invulnerable to unforeseen events.

Third significant factor, one of the responding officers had a teenage daughter who attempted suicide the year before. While his daughter had been in treatment and was reportedly stable, witnessing the death of this young boy brought up many of the feelings he had when his own child had attempted suicide. He had been the one to find her unconscious body. Fortunately, in his case, his daughter survived. Yet, as any parent or person who has ever had a family member attempt suicide knows, sometimes ones grasp on reality can be fragile and fleeting. No parent ever expects their child to die before them, especially in a suicide. If it happened once, could it happen again?

As can almost be expected when working with emergency public safety professionals, not one of the officers confided in the other about their feelings, but they openly shared their feelings with me. The Watch Commander, a female Sergeant with 18 years on the job, didn't wait for them to come to her. She knew the circumstances of the death, made a reasonable prediction about the impact the death would have on her officers, and knowing a little bit about the circumstances concerning Officer "Smith's" daughter made the decision to call me in.

She didn't have to do anything, if she didn't want to, but she decided to work proactively and preventatively. She took the extra step. Later, she also checked in with her officers individually when they returned on their next duty day. No big song and dance, no standing on soapboxes for an oratory speech, no lengthy extended appointment to discuss deep-seated psychological problems. Just a few words said at the right time and at the right place, "Just checking in with you. How's it going?"

A simple act of genuine concern towards an individual can do so much to preserve the integrity and safety of a professional relationship and working environment. Ultimately, everyone benefits, including the organization.

Family Members, Partners, Friends, Parents of EPSP

"Unless you're one of us you can't possibly understand what it's like to be one of us. The things we see and experience every day... how can we even begin to explain them to you?"

A common explanation, and inarguably the truth: How does one assess the severity of the circumstances surrounding the needs of the person you love? With diligence, perseverance and patience. There is a fine line, at times, between what you need to know and what you want to know. Certainly there are some circumstances that your partner (family member, friend, etc) in EPSP can not share with you that are duty related, however, the feelings associated with their experiences can always be shared. Are you ready to listen?

A Young Couple

The other month I was with a young couple, married for five years, and an officer for six. The officer was a first responder on a "jumper" (a suicide by jumping off a 14 story building). It had been his first time responding to a completed suicide in which the injuries were so catastrophic. He was extremely upset but maintained throughout the call.

Once the coroner had removed the body he'd returned to the division to complete his paperwork on the incident, and called his wife. His wife wanted to listen to him, but when he began to describe the details of the injuries his wife stopped him. Later, she was angry with him for telling her such terrible things. He stopped talking to her about most things related to work.

Two years later, I saw them in marital counseling. In session with me she complained that he never talked to her about anything anymore. She felt disregarded and detached. He complained that he never knew what was safe and what wasn't safe to talk about. Rather then upset her because he did love her, he simply "sucked it up" and stopped talking.

"I didn't feel comfortable talking in a group with my peers so I didn't. I tried to talk to my wife about it but she couldn't listen. I talked to a couple female co-workers about it but that only made it worse, so I continued to repress my feelings. I had flashbacks and nightmares on and off for almost two years. I told no one."

Finding and seeing the body at the scene is the single strongest predictor of grief severity. In Predictors and Correlates of Grief and Suicide researcher Jay Callahan recommends that support groups need to pay attention to the trauma of suicide as well as the grief reactions, including helping people talk about and cope with traumatic images.

Those of you who are emotionally involved with someone in emergency public safety are in a tenuous position. Like the woman I just described to you, you may not want to hear the gory details about what your partner sees or listens to every day, but you don't have to hear the gory details to be emotionally present for someone you care about. All you really have to do is be there and show up for the experience. What you will then be privileged to listen to is some very important information about someone you care deeply about.

People working in emergency public safety are repeatedly exposed to suicide and death. It is, unfortunately, a routine part of their job. Some EPS professionals can become exceedingly proficient at denying the presence of their own feelings, yet they are still impacted by their experiences everyday. There is no hard and fast rule as to when and what will tip the barrel and open the floodgates for any one individual. Everyone is different and their tolerance level, history and personal experiences will influence their response and reactions to any single or series of events, but if Red Flags are coming up on the horizon for you concerning the person you love, don't ignore them. The Red Flags are there for a reason.

You may also be inclined to believe that because your loved one is not on the front line, he or she is a 911 dispatcher; you don't have to

be concerned. Wrong. I know few dispatchers who do not feel they are first on scene when responding to a call. In fact, the vast majority of dispatchers I've worked with feel that as a First Point of Contact they are as much on scene of an event as a First Responder. Unfortunately dispatchers receive about half the recognition or validation as First Responders do while experiencing relatively equivalent levels of stress and trauma related to the calls they handle. Ultimately it has an impact.

"I took a 911 call from a woman whose husband was having a difficult time breathing. Easy enough, I thought, or maybe the word is "routine." We started going through E.M.D. and some prearrivals. The call progressively got worse. The man stopped breathing and I instructed the woman to do CPR. As she was performing CPR she was relaying the fact that her husband had lung cancer. He didn't make it.

The rescue squad that arrived on scene relayed the information to me later on. I wished I had never been told.

The Fire Chief was the first to arrive on scene. He found the entryway, where the man had collapsed, completely covered in blood. He said he had never in his entire career seen anything like it. He slipped in the blood on the floor. The patient was covered in it. The wife was covered from head to foot in blood, the walls, etc. I think you get the picture. Basically, his lungs and most of his blood were in the entryway or covering his wife.

I was very insistent with her that we do CPR and that she not stop until the rescue squad arrived. I feel responsible for the last moments she spent with her husband; the last memory she will have of him, and the fact that she was left with all that blood and tissue to clean up off of herself and her clothing.

This call never seems to go away."

Love An EPS Professional?

Then Next Time You Sit Down To Talk, Remember The Nitty Gritty

- Take the time to ask.
- Be willing to hear the answer.
- Be open with your concerns.
- Share your own feelings.
- Let them know how much you value him or her.
- Be available to talk about it again later.
- Don't judge.
- Don't criticize.
- Don't humiliate or induce guilt.
- It's not about you.
- It isn't personal.

STILL UNCOMFORTABLE ?

If you're still not sure of what you've heard, or you are unable to feel satisfied, calmed or comfortable with the responses provided (be excruciatingly honest with yourself here), **take the next step**. Talk to someone outside of the relationship, either to a trusted friend or family member, clergy or to a professional, either alone or with your partner in tow. I call it, "Getting a reality check." Your partner may become angry, emotional or irritated by your actions, but consider the alternative.

I have rolled out to far too many suicides of emergency public safety professionals and in almost every case the individual gave signs of his or her intent in the weeks preceding the suicide.

You may not want to hear it, you may not want to see it but if you're feeling it and seeing a behavioral and emotional change, it's there. Trust the feeling. It may not be as bad or as serious as you are fearful of, but if you don't ask; if you don't look to see what's really going on you may not find out until it's too late. Mark Twain said it best: "Da-nile ain't just a river in Egypt."

"Oh Say Can You See, The Red Flags Flying Over Me."

For those of you who want, or need, more.

You're reading this section because you endorsed one or more of the following sections on the List of 16: 5, 6, 11, 12 or 13 with Plane Crash, Bombing or PDVF with Children, giving you an automatic Four Red Flags. You may wonder why we are weighing these experiences so heavily, particularly if you believe that you have come a long way from those early experiences, perhaps occurring during childhood, and now as an adult you've "put all that behind you and moved on." This may be true.

Other experiences may be more recent and are ones that may have occurred to you as an adult or on the job. As an emergency public safety professional it is hard not to have come into direct contact with any number of extraordinary circumstances, some of which, if you work for a large urban organization, become almost standard fare to the EPS professional. Suicides, homicides, child abuse, and domestic violence all come with the territory, and we almost become "numb" to them. We handled them a hundred times before and we'll handle them a hundred times again before our career comes to a close.

Then, there are some of you who were reluctant to endorse any items because you already knew the list was far longer then you really wanted to acknowledge. Like many good men and women I've met in my practice, and in my life, when I ask you how long you've been depressed, you answer, "I don't know. Seems like I've always felt this way."

My intention in flagging these items is not to dispute the quality of your mental health or the prowess by which you have healed and moved on from painful experiences in your life. My intention is to highlight that there are some experiences that occur in our lives that undeniably change who we are as people, and because of those experiences we will never look at the world the same again.

Like many things, this in itself does not have to be an obstacle to living your life or doing your job, as long as you have an awareness of what belongs to you and your history and feelings, and what belongs to the other person and or situation. This is particularly important when working and making decisions in your capacity as an EPS professional.

Sergeant North

I met Sergeant North after he transferred to a new division of a large metropolitan police department. Tall, strikingly handsome, well respected and admired for his work as a professional Sgt. North was said to bc on the fast track to success and promotion on the department. Yet, there was a side to Sgt North that few people saw, on or off the job. His personal life was a shambles.

I met him after the dissolution of yet another relationship with a beautiful woman whom he characterized as chaotic, destructive and "high drama." On several occasions the conflicts in his relationships escalated to the point of violence, with injuries, and on one occasion an outside agency was called to intervene.

It was with great hesitancy and shame Sgt. North admitted that he was the repeated victim of domestic violence. He never fought back. He was depressed and had been depressed for as long as he could remember. The only period of time in his life that he could remember feeling happy was his first year with the department, while in the academy. Shortly after graduating and while still on his probation, his troubles began with his first girlfriend. His personal life had yet to turn around.

One of four children Sgt North left home at the age of 16 to move in with friends and finish high school. His dream was to become a police officer. His father was a physically abusive tyrant who was both drug and alcohol addicted. His mother was a passive, emotionally fragile woman who eventually broke under the strain of the physical abuse she endured from his father.

Sgt North's home as a child was frequently the scene of loud dramatic fighting, and horrific and unpredictable violence. On more than one occasion the police were called to respond to reports of domestic violence that many times led to the arrest and incarceration of his father, a former Viet Nam Veteran.

Sgt North left home as soon as he was old enough and at his first legal opportunity. He went on to graduate high school and then immediately applied to a law enforcement agency out of state. He was accepted into the Police Academy. It was his dreams come true. After graduating he went on to become a highly decorated police officer and eventually promoted.

On the job he was a stellar performer. Off the job he was depressed, disillusioned, often despondent and frequently suicidal. He was resigned to live a life that he believed would never match up to what he had once hoped for. He never told anyone on the job how he actually felt and believed that it had no impact whatsoever on his work performance.

"Why," he asked, "do I always seem to end up with women who are hell bent on destroying me? I do everything for them. I support them. I give them anything they want. I never argue. I don't drink. I don't smoke. I don't cheat. I'm reasonably good looking. When they hit me I never even fight back. I swore I'd never be like my father. But, in the end nothing seems to matter. They still leave me, and they blame me for the problems!"

How does an attractive bright police officer with all the ear markings for success end up the depressed despondent victim of domestic violence? As a law enforcement officer he'd successfully responded to countless incidents of domestic violence and prided himself on his ability to resolve issues without force. As a supervisor and Sergeant he'd counseled numerous trainees and probationers on marital and relationship issues, and had even become a peer counselor to improve his skills. Yet, in his own personal life he was unable to function.

Is this just one person out of a million? No, in fact the disparity between home life and personal is far more common then you would think. I have met countless good men and women who are consummate professionals and yet, in their personal lives there are huge gaps.

On more then one occasion I've asked a client, "Does your family background and history have any impact on who you are as a professional or how you do business?" In most instances the answer is a resounding, "No." Some will say, "It's because of what I went through as a child that I became a police officer," or dispatcher, or EMT, but few will admit that personal experiences they've had either on the job or off have profoundly influenced them professionally.

Sgt North may want to believe that his family history, or his history with women and failed relationships, does not impact how he does business as a police officer and supervisor, but he would be wrong.

No one lives in a vacuum. In his case he learned early on that his "job," so to speak, was about tolerating and enduring abusive relationships. His threshold for tolerating dysfunctional behavior was much higher then many of his colleagues.

In some cases this proved to be an advantage in that he was more willing to hang in there with a problematic probationer who was "higher maintenance" than other probationers because he believed that in the end he or she could still make a great officer. However in other cases for Sgt North, it was a potential liability. That same ability to tolerate highly dysfunctional behavior also made him vulnerable to **not** seeing certain types of warning signs or Red Flags concerning particular types of probationers, or other officers. Often times it was not until the problem behavior became so flagrant that it was undeniable. He became forced by circumstances to respond. This left him, at times, in a perilous position, and he did not always make the best choice.

This same process played out in his personal life as well. Every time he picked someone new he believed he was picking someone who was nothing like the last woman he was involved with. Yet, each time the relationship ultimately bore a striking similarity to the last and with it all of the same resultant problems. In each case, it was also not until the relationship became a high stakes high drama that the women in his life were able to get his attention, but by then it was usually too late.

He always seemed to be the last one to know, on each occasion, that this would happen.

So, what does this mean in the final analysis?

It means that Sgt North has certain vulnerabilities that are derived from his life experiences. In his case, starting with his childhood that became further complicated by his experiences as an adult and as a police officer. As long as Sgt North continues to live with a certain amount of denial he will feed those vulnerabilities, and he will probably continue to be surprised when the next woman he picks turns out to be just like the last woman he picked, again.

For most of us who are relatively high functioning the work place is usually the last place that is affected. The manifestation of his vulnerability at work may not be as dramatic as it was with his past lovers, but eventually it will manifest in his professional life. It only takes one time to miss something important in public safety and inadvertently place someone at risk.

Is there no hope for Sgt North? Of course there's hope. There's always hope if you are willing to look with both eyes open.

Life is unavoidable. The good and the bad, everything about who you are and what you have experienced has gone into who you are as an adult, and as a professional. Even your experiences as a child, as the caretaker of your woefully neglectful parent, have contributed to the adult you grew up to be. It was all part of your path, and whether you are consciously aware of this or not, it has contributed to why you chose a helping profession to begin with.

As a psychologist I have to be aware of what belongs to me and what belongs to other people. It's my job. If I am unable to distinguish the difference and I over identify with a client then I'm in trouble and ultimately the therapy is in trouble. My job is to be aware of where the lines are.

As a supervisor, training officer, Watch Commander, Shift Supervisor, police officer, EMT, dispatcher, we are all inherently tasked with knowing where the lines are. Few of us come from perfect backgrounds or have lives that haven't in some way been touched by tragic or painful circumstances, but that does not in itself have to become an obstacle to living our lives unless we choose it to be that way. Sgt North didn't intend on becoming a victim in his life. He looked like anything but a victim on the surface, but many of his choices have pulled him down that path. Until now, he has not wanted to take responsibility for what is his life.

I didn't have an idyllic childhood. I've had experiences that at times have separated me from those of others, and I haven't always wanted to see the part I've played in creating the problems or maintaining the dysfunctional behavior, but there came a point when I decided I'd had enough.

As a psychologist I've believed it was also my professional obligation to be willing to look at what is mine and to do the work needed to become healthier. I have come to understand, accept and take responsibility for what is my life. I've learned how to use these experiences to inform me about what is really important to me and what choices I need to make. I'm not always right. I still make mistakes, but that's OK. I'm human and as long as I'm willing to be abundantly clear and painfully honest with myself, when I need to be, and sometimes even when I don't want to be, it works out. I have a good life and I am able to do my job, and do it well.

I've come to accept that I cannot treat every person who comes to me for help, no matter how much they may want me to, and that I may not always be the best fit for every situation I am asked to handle. I know now I don't have to. My responsibility is knowing when to say "No," and when to refer out.

Everything about my life, my experiences in my family, my friends, the way kids used to tease me in elementary school for being "too tall and having curly hair," the day my mother died, the year we lost our house, the first time a boy ever kissed me, (His name was Mike and we were standing in the stationhouse of the Long Island Rail Road in Kings Park. I was in eighth grade. My mother drove up just as his lips touched mine.), to my experiences as an adult, the first suicide I ever witnessed, the first time my heart was broken, the first moment I saw the lifeless body of the bank robber at my feet at the scene of the North Hollywood Bank Robbery of 1997, all of these experiences and feelings have gone into who I am and have made me the adult, the person and the clinician that I am.

This is neither good nor bad. It's just what it is, my life as I know it, the same as yours is for you.

We all have Red Flags. The challenge is being honest with ourselves. If you're not the person for the situation, if you're too close to the person you're concerned about, if your own feelings are getting in the way and clouding your judgment, there's no shame to this as long as you are aware of your potential vulnerabilities or Red Flags. With awareness we have choices. With denial we have only reactions and sometimes the decisions are made for us. When that happens, sometimes there's no going back again.

Organizations, Books, Articles, Websites and Other Resources

ARTICLES

Psychosocial Approaches to Suicide Prevention: Applications to Patients with Bipolar Disorders, Gray SM, Otto MW; Journal of Clinical Psychiatry 2001; 62 Suppl 25: 56-64

Pharmacologic Interventions in Suicide Prevention, Tondo L, Ghiani C, Albert M; Journal of Clinical Psychiatry 2001; 62 Suppl 25: 51-55

Childhood abuse, household dysfunction and risk of attempted suicide throughout the life span: findings from Adverse Childhood Experiences study, Dube SR, Anda RF, Felitti VS, Chapman DP, Williamson DF, Gibs WH; Journal of American Medical Association 2001 Dec 26; 286 (24) 3126-3127

Coping, meaning in life, and suicidal manifestations: examining gender differences, Edwards MJ, Holden RR; Journal of Clinical Psychology 2001 Dec; 57 (12) 1517-1534

The National Strategy for Suicide Prevention Krulewitch CJ; Journal of Midwifery Womens Health 2001 Sep-Oct, 46 (5) 304

Training Program in suicide prevention for psychiatric nursing personnel enhance attitudes to attempted suicide patients, Samuelsson M, Asbey M,; International Journal of Nursing Studies, Vol 39, Issue 1 Jan 2002 115-121

What would you say to the person on the roof? A Suicide Prevention Text, Elitzur AC, Omer H; Suicide Life Threat Behavior 2001 Summer, 31 (2) 129-139

Recognizing and Responding to a Suicide Crisis, Hendin H, Maltzberger JT, Lipschitz A, Haas AP, Kyle J; Ann N.Y. Acad Sci 2001 Apr, 932: 169-186

Therapists' Reactions to Patients' Suicides American Journal of Psychiatry 2000 Dec, 157 (12): 2022-2027

A New Suicide, Bhalerao S; Journal of Family Practice 2001 June; 50 (6): 551

Developing a comprehensive school suicide prevention program, King KA; Journal of School Health 2001 Apr; 71 (4) 132-137

Suicide Prevention. Holding On
Laurent C; Health Services Journal 2000 Oct 5; 110 (5725): Suppl 6-7

Preventing Suicide and Premature Death by Education and Treatment, Rutz W; Journal of Affective Disorders 2001 Jan; 62 (1-2) 123-129

From the Centers for Disease Control and Prevention: Suicide Prevention Among Active Duty Air Force Personnel–United States 1990-1999; Journal of the American Medical Association 2000 Jan 12; 283 (2): 193-194

A Review of the Literature On Prevention of Suicide Through Interventions in Accident and Emergency Departments, Repper J; Journal of Clinical Nursing 1999 Jan; 8 (1): 3-12

Suicide Prevention Protocol, Robie D, Edgemon-Hill EJ, Phelps B, Schmitz C, Laughlin JA; American Journal of Nursing 99 Dec; 99 (12): 53-55, 57

A Suicide Prevention Advisory Group at an Academic Medical Center, Hough D, Lewis P; Military Medicine 2000 Feb; 165 (2): 97-100

Adolescent Victimization and Associated Suicidal and Violent Behavior Cleary SD; Adolescence 2000 Winter; 35 (140): 671-682

Effects of Different Telephone Intervention Styles with Suicide Callers at Two Suicide Prevention Centers: An Empirical Investigation, Mishara BL, Daigle MS; American Journal of Community Psychology 1997 Dec; 25 (6): 861-885

Suicide Prevention Plan Calls for Physicians' Help, Vastag B; Journal of the American Medical Association 2001 Jun 6; 285 (21): 2701-2703

Evaluation of Indicated Suicide Risk Prevention Approaches for Potential High School Dropouts, Thompson EA, Eggert LL, Randall BP, Pike KL; American Journal of Public Health 2001 May; 91 (5): 742-752

WEB SITES

http://www.suicideprevention.com
http://www.webmd.com
http://www.acpm.org (American College of Preventive Medicine)
http://www.jfponline.com (Journal of Family Practice)
http://www.suicideinfo.ca/siec

OTHER RESOURCES:

Suicide Prevention Forum

American Association of Suicidology

Suicide Prevention Centers (nation-wide)

Suicide Prevention Hotline (available in most states)

American Foundation for Suicide Prevention

Surgeon General Releases Suicide-Prevention Strategy, Sean Martin May 2, 2001

Buying a Handgun Significantly Increases Risk of Suicide, Peggy Peck 17 Nov 1999

Anger: The Fifth Food Group

WHEN RAGE BECOMES A WAY OF LIFE

Chapter 2

Anger: The Fifth Food Group

WHEN RAGE BECOMES A WAY OF LIFE

"If you really want to be in law enforcement be prepared to constantly be challenged with balancing your life professionally. If you're not good at balancing, seriously rethink your career choice. This job becomes a way of life."

The first time I wrote about anger I was motivated by my work with dispatchers. The Angry Dispatcher: Fact or Fiction remains the most requested article on dr911.com, to date. Since it's original publication much has changed in the EPS community and as many public safety agencies across the country lurch through sometimes tumultuous, too often painful transitions, the personal and professional lives of those who continue the work are dramatically impacted.

From the physical and health implications of unresolved anger to the unfortunate manifestations of anger we bear witness to on the road, in the workplace, on the schoolyard and at home, anger is fast becoming one of society's greatest concerns and most significant problems.

This chapter attempts to address these unprecedented changes in emergency public safety and the far ranging impact on its members. We will review the facts about anger and its health implications, touch on the personal impact it has on the home front and with the family, and offer suggestions for understanding as well as tools for coping.

Those of you who would like to read the original article entitled The Angry Dispatcher: Fact or Fiction will find it located in Appendix 1.

Big News Flash: Times Have Changed

It doesn't take a rocket scientist to know, "Toto, we're not in Kansas anymore." Regardless of your rank, job title or employment classification the everyday workplace has changed, and with it the way many professionals are asked to do business.

Much of what you may remember as a recruit, trainee or new employee bears little resemblance to what we see now.

Not unlike corporate America, public legislation and private litigation have transformed the organizational climate, forcing even the secular world of emergency public safety to change.

As can be expected not all changes have gone smoothly, or with regard for its employees. Were we only discussing those responsible for the management of paperclips the transitions might be more palatable to those who must bear the brunt of the changes, but the grim reality is we're not. We are talking about people whose everyday work life is rarely mundane.

The everyday uncertainty regarding life and death, and how close any one of us comes to that invisible line during the course of our workday has a way of bringing even the most minor event into the most extraordinary focus.

In The Broadest Sense

Everyday our senses are flooded with the violence perpetrated by others. The news media, popular television and movies are quick to remind us of the full gamut of human potential, both positive and negative.

For those of us tasked with providing the emergency response to humanities frightening expressions of self, we rarely need the media to serve as a reminder. One day on the job alone is enough to refresh our memories of the horrors people are more than capable of. We see it, hear it and even smell it on any given day we decide to show up for work. We may turn off the television or discontinue the newspaper subscription but the memories are never far from recall.

But is this the only source of our stress? In a random sample of police officers participating in an ongoing research study (Chace, 2001), 4 out of 5 identified work place factors (such as problems with supervisors, and pending complaints) as the primary source of their stress, and consequent anger and frustration.

> "I can deal with emergencies. I can't handle idiot co-workers and radios that don't work and dispatch procedures conceived by idiots!"

The Every Day Reality

How easy if the only threat we managed every day was the one we encountered on the street or over the air. How freeing to know that once we hung up the gun belt, took off the headset, turned in the keys, or took off the uniform, life was immeasurably better because we knew at the end of the day it was a job well done: To be supported and rewarded by our organization, treated with respect by our supervisors and colleagues, appreciated by the public we served and loved unconditionally by our friends and family around us; what a wonderful world that would be.

Few would argue if that were the world most people lived and worked in, but how many of us can say that? What happened?

From The Worried Well to Managing Risk

Even as a psychologist, things have changed. In the beginning of my career the worst situation I generally encountered in my office were tearful and distraught individuals who were unhappy with some aspect of their lives. Occasionally someone expressed suicidal ideation but rarely did someone present with active psychotic symptoms or florid homicidal intent. The vast majority of people I treated were easily categorized as "the worried well;" people who were generally content with their lot in life, functioning fairly well overall but felt some anxiety in specific areas of their lives.

Then a subtle shift occurred and my practice went from treating the worried well to conducting threat assessments on people that rarely looked any different then you or I but were described as "dangerous," "threatening" and "volatile."

Conducting threat assessments are now routine for most practitioners, and while the "worried well" still find their way to my office, the potential risk factors I'm forced to consider when I'm sitting with someone are staggering.

Developing systems for evaluating dangerousness has become an extremely lucrative and necessary business but despite elaborate schemes for determining risk factors people are still dying at the hands of others with alarming regularity.

Grimly we are reminded that systems of evaluation are helpful but offer no guarantees. No one has a crystal ball and regardless of what your technique or method we are not always able to see what can't be seen.

No matter what you may think you're heard there really isn't any exact way to predict someone's behavior, and the range, intensity and frequency of individuals acting out aggressively in the work place and at home continues to hit new highs.

"If you want people to like you, become a fireman. Don't become a cop. Nobody likes cops."

THE OFFICERS AND CIVILIANS I SEE and come into contact with are angry and frustrated, not only with the changes that have occurred organizationally, but also with public perception of the job they do. Morale, for many, is at an all time low, and everybody knows it. But who is doing anything about it?

On more then one occasion I have listened to the anger and frustration vented by officers towards the department. I've heard discussions of the inevitability of workplace violence perpetrated by one of their own toward command staff as though it were already a foregone conclusion; it wasn't a question of if but rather when, where and who.

This isn't just one isolated incident in a department nobody knows. Agencies all over the country are creating training protocols for handling the eventuality of such an event, and again, the general consensus is, 'We're not training for whether it will happen. We're training for when it will happen.'

Not all my experiences have been from my position as an "armchair general." I've been the witness to and the unwitting recipient of workplace and organizational practices and behaviors that have left me angry, and disheartened by the very process that is theoretically designed to protect its recipients.

I have listened to the willful distortion of truth, the deliberate manipulation of facts and the blatant disregard for the value of others by people who 'should' know better by virtue of their position and authority, and yet choose not to see because to do so would not be in the best interest of those empowered.

"People keep talking about the department like it's this living entity, and nothing else matters. It's as though there really aren't any people who work there, it's just "The Department. That's it. Everyone else is expendable as long as 'The Department' keeps going."

It is with good reason people are angry, and as one paramedic shared, after her exposure to a homeless indigent infested with ticks left her with Lymes Disease:

"I was cursed at, yelled at, humiliated at times in front of others by my partner and a few lieutenants. One lieutenant almost hit me in the face with a metal transaction splint."

Some current practices in the workplace simply don't make sense, and it doesn't seem to be getting any easier.

Nationally

More and more Americans are feeling pushed to the breaking point. The American Automobile Association's Foundation for Traffic Safety says incidents of violently aggressive driving- which some dub "mad driver disease" rose 7% a year in the '90s.

Airlines are reporting more outbursts of sky rage. And sideline rage has become widespread: A Pennsylvania kids' football game ended in a brawl involving more than 100 coaches, players, parents and fans. In a particularly tragic incident that captured national attention, a Massachusetts father- angered over rough play during his son's hockey practice- beat another father to death as their children watched.

No one seems immune to the anger epidemic. Women fly off the handle just as often as men, though they are less likely to get physical. Young people may seem more volatile, but even senior citizens have erupted into "line rage" and pushed ahead of others simply because they felt they had "waited long enough" in their lives.

Violent outbursts are just as likely to occur in the suburbs as they are in the city. "Everyone seems to be hotter under the collar these days," said Sybil Evans, a conflict resolution expert in New York City, who singles out three primary culprits: time, technology and tension. "Americans are working longer hours than anyone else in the world. The cell phones and pagers that were supposed to make our lives easier have put us on call 24/7/365. Since we're always running, we're tense and low on patience. And the less patience we have, the less we monitor what we say to people and how we treat them."

Ironically, the fluctuations in our economy seem to have brought out the worst in some people. "Never have so many people with so much been so unhappy," offers Leslie Charles, author of *Why Is Everyone So Cranky*? "There are more of us than ever before, all wanting the same space, goods, toys, services or attention. Everyone thinks, 'me first. I don't have time to be polite.' We've lost not only our civility but all tolerance for inconvenience."

The sheer complexity of our lives has also shortened our fuse. We rely on computers that crash, cell phones that die, drive on roads that gridlock, and place calls to machines that put us on endless hold. "Its not any one thing but lots of little things that make people feel like they don't have control of their lives," says Jane Middleton-Moz, a therapist and author. "A sense of helplessness is what triggers rage. Its why people end up kicking ATM machines."

Is It In The Blood?

"People no longer hold themselves accountable for bad behavior," says Doris Wide Helmering, a therapist and author of Sense Ability. "They blame anyone and everything for their anger."

Survival

When the sales clerk wouldn't accept the return and give his girlfriend her money back, an Arizona dispatcher became so enraged he ripped the cash register off the counter and threw it across the store. Playing golf, he sometimes became so angry that he threw his clubs 50 feet up the fairway and into the trees and had to get someone to retrieve them. Arguments with his girlfriend usually ended when he pitched most of her belongings out the second story window of their home. He was suspended from work and ordered into anger management classes.

While some people may seem like they were born angry, few rarely are. As adults they may appear to thrive on conflict and chaos, and may even go out of their way to create it, but as children it is unlikely they started out this way.

Anger as a filter through which we see and respond to the world is usually learned behavior. As is the case for most defense mechanisms, in the beginning there was a legitimate reason for their existence. Parents who neglect us, siblings who pick on us, circumstances that overwhelm us; defense mechanisms develop as a means towards helping us cope with our feelings. As more primitive defense mechanisms, (such as blocking and projection), outlive their usefulness they are replaced by more sophisticated defense mechanisms, (such as humor and intellectualization.) With "luck" and good intention we learn from our mistakes.

Many people end up in my office after they've insisted on "knocking their heads against the wall" a couple hundred times. They're adults, they're professionals, and this is the way they've always done things. This is also the way they want to keep doing things, but despite their best efforts it doesn't seem to work anymore! Anger is typically one of the problems identified. They're locked into their worldview and they don't want to change. Give them half a chance and they'll vent to anyone who will listen but even after doing so nothing seems to get any better.

Venting may make you feel better right now, but it only lasts for a moment. "Catharsis is worse than useless," says Brad Bushman, a psychology professor at Iowa State University whose research has shown that letting anger out makes people more aggressive, not less. "Many people think of anger as the psychological equivalent of the steam in a pressure cooker: It has to be released, or it will explode. That's not true. The people who react by hitting, kicking, screaming and swearing just feel more angry."

"You Can't Make Me!"

The destructive effects of anger are well documented. People who are anger prone are much more likely to develop heart disease.

Study after study demonstrate that anger, rage and hostility are particularly damaging to the cardiovascular system and a major risk factor in heart disease at least equal to or perhaps even greater then traditionally recognized risk factors such as high cholesterol and high blood pressure. And for the first time, a study demonstrated a link between how easily a person is angered and early signs of heart disease in young adults.

In a ground breaking study, 374 men and women ages 18-30 were followed over ten years to determine the factors that might predict the development of coronary heart disease in later life. At the start of the study they completed a 50-item, true false questionnaire designed to measure how often a person becomes angry, how mistrustful a person is, and how aggressive the anger makes them. For example: "I think most people would lie to get ahead." "It's safer to trust nobody." "No one cares much what happens to you." "I have at times had to be rough with people who were rude to me."

Ten years later the same people had a noninvasive heart scan that measured the amount of calcium in the walls of coronary arteries, a sign of early atherosclerosis (narrowing of the arteries). Those with the highest hostility scores were twice as likely to have measurable calcification of the arteries. The damaging association with hostility persisted even after controlling for age, gender, smoking, body weight, cholesterol and blood pressure. The thirteen volunteers with the highest scores on the hostility test were nine times more likely to have evidence of early atherosclerosis compared to the lowest anger group.

In another recent study of 13,000 middle-aged men and women, anger-prone people had 2-3 times the incidence of heart attacks, bypass surgery and balloon angioplasty. In this study, anger was measured with a 10-question survey (see Anger Self-Test).

Results

Eight percent scored in the high-trait anger range, fifty-five percent in the moderate range and thirty-seven percent in the low range. The high-anger subjects with normal blood pressure levels were at much greater risk of heart disease including a fatal heart attack. Interestingly, those people with high blood pressure did not have an increased risk due to anger. One reason may be that those with high blood pressure were taking medications that not only lowers blood pressure but also blunts the harmful effects of anger.

ANGER SELF TEST	*ALMOST NEVER*	*SOMETIMES*	*OFTEN*	*ALMOST ALWAYS*
I am quick tempered.	1	2	3	4
I have a fiery temper.	1	2	3	4
I am a hotheaded person	1	2	3	4
I get angry when I am slowed down by other's mistakes.	1	2	3	4
I feel annoyed when I am not given recognition for doing good work.	1	2	3	4
I fly off the handle.	1	2	3	4
When I get angry, I say nasty things.	1	2	3	4
It makes me furious when I am criticized in front of others.	1	2	3	4
When I get angry I feel like hitting someone.	1	2	3	4

Anger Self-Test

Circle your response for each item, and then add up the total for all items.
10-14 = low anger 15-21 = moderate anger 22-36 = high anger

How does hostility harm the heart? Several pathways have been suggested. Hostile people tend to release more stress hormones that can cause blood pressure to surge, heart rhythms to disrupt, and blood platelets to clot blocking an artery.

Fortunately we can learn to diffuse anger and change hostile patterns of behavior, thoughts, feelings and actions. Patients who have had heart attacks can reduce their risk of recurrence by as much as 50% by learning anger management and relaxation skills and getting social support.

Emergency Public Safety and Anger

Diffusing anger and changing patterns may be easily accomplished at home with friends and family, or in a controlled study, but how possible is this in emergency public safety when much of what we come into contact with is outside of our control?

Learning to effectively managing anger on the job is challenging, but it is not impossible. Like that old bad joke about psychologists: How many psychologists does it take to change a light bulb? One, but it has to want to change.

The Facts

The pressure on personnel in public safety is enormous and the resultant stress has struck broadly across every rank, level, size and type of organization nationwide. Trained professionals everywhere are leaving their chosen careers and jobs faster then employers can replace them. In law enforcement alone, officers are leaving large once prestigious metropolitan police agencies for smaller agencies, or leaving law enforcement entirely, in unprecedented numbers.

Organizations once considered the pride of policing are in desperate trouble, unable to hold on to tenured officers, and yet unable to successfully recruit new ones. In Los Angeles, where the police have been buffeted with scandal since the Rodney King beating in 1991, there were only 19 recruits in the police academy class in June of 2001. In July Los Angeles canceled the police academy classes because there not enough recruits. Retired officers were offered attractive financial incentives to return to the fold while specialized divisions were dissolved, its staff returned to the streets to work patrol in an effort to find enough warm bodies to police the city.

The New York Times reported that police departments across the nation are facing what some call a personnel crisis, with the number of recruits at record lows, an increasing number of experienced officers turning down promotions to sergeant or lieutenant and many talented senior officers declining offers to become police chiefs, executive recruiters and police officials say.

These problems have come at a time when crime is at its lowest levels since the late 1960's and morale should be high. But, the experts say, many officers from the lowest to the highest rank are questioning their occupation, tempted by higher pay in the private sector after a decade long economic boom and discouraged by seemingly constant public and news criticism about police brutality and racial profiling.

"When I look at the job I do and what I have done over the years, specifically the last few years, I find it difficult to swallow that jagged little pill. It's very easy to continue to move through this career on its proverbial 'roller coaster,' but its not until one really looks at all the 'stuff' they've dealt with that it becomes REAL."

There are no nationwide statistics on the problem. But figures from several cities show the magnitude of the drop in applicants for the police examination, the first step to becoming a police officer. In Chicago last year, 5,263 people signed up for the exam, despite months of recruiting at college campuses, military bases and churches throughout the Midwest, said Cmdr. Bill Powers, the head of the Chicago police personnel division. That is down from 10,290 people who signed up in 1997 and 36,211 applicants in 1991. Traditionally, only a small fraction who apply are eventually accepted making a large applicant pool especially important.

In New York City, more than 1,700 officers left the 41,000 member force last year through retirement or resignation, a third more then the year before. The retirement rate is expected to accelerate with concerns about morale and pay taking their toll and with a large portion of the force soon to complete 20 years of service, when officers can retire with a full pension.

The number of captains leaving the New York City Police department tripled in the 2000 fiscal year from the year before, and over the next four years, more than half of the force's 2,100 captains and lieutenants will be eligible to retire.

In Seattle, the police department is having trouble finding officers to take the sergeants' examination, and sergeants to take the exam for promotion to lieutenant. Only 86 officers took this years sergeants exam, down from 134 in 1997, and only 10 sergeants took this years' exam for lieutenant, compared with 33 in 1997, department figures show.

Many officers with seniority do not want to start over in a higher rank, risking having to work weekends, officers say. And some sergeants do not want the promotion because lieutenants, unlike sergeants, do not get overtime pay.

"So why would a detective want to give up that work schedule when they have a family," he asked, "in order to be a lieutenant without seniority and face working nights and week ends?"

Attrition is a growing problem from New York to Los Angeles. In Detroit, where the police department is under a federal investigation for charges that the police routinely violated citizens' civil rights, 600 to 700 officers have resigned in the last five years, many to take better-paying jobs in suburban forces. In addition, more than 1,000 other officers have retired in the last five years, and 1,000 more are eligible to retire in the next two years, a large proportion of Detroit's 4,000-member department.

Low pay is often a factor. In Detroit, the starting salary for a police officer is $28,865; in Houston, it is $26,000.

In Miami, the police department has only 883 officers; well below it's authorized strength of 1,045 officers. "Because of the economy, people are not really interested in law enforcement as a career," said Sgt. David Ramras of the Miami police-recruiting unit.

Sgt. John Rivera, the president of the Miami-Dade Police Benevolent Association, offered another explanation. "This is increasingly becoming a more miserable job by the day," Sergeant Rivera said. It has not helped, he said, that the Miami police have been stung by accusations of abuse, corruption and cover-ups, and the department is under investigation by federal prosecutors.

Most officers are good people, he said, "so to risk your life for increasingly ungrateful people isn't worth it."

Mr. Oldani, president of the Oldani Group, an executive search firm in Bellevue, Washington, offered this example. Last month, Chief Kerlikowske went out for a run from police headquarters and came across a crowd surrounding a woman who had passed out- from a heroin overdose, it turned out. The chief, in his jogging gear, stopped to give her mouth-to-mouth resuscitation, then, when she began to breathe again, took her to the hospital. Later, Chief Kerlikowske had to go to the hospital himself, for hepatitis B shots.

But, on the evening news, Mr. Oldani said, the chief's good deed merited just a few seconds. The major item, he said, was about the police chase of a stolen car, which struck a pedestrian, and the criticism that the police were to blame for the injured pedestrian.

"It's a good example of what's wrong," Mr. Oldani said. "He was being a good cop, and that just got lost."

Today's Climate

"There's been a big change in the culture of policing in the past few years, as lifestyle becomes more important then the sense of public service," said Carroll Buracker, the head of a management and consulting firm in Harrisburg, Va., and a former police chief in Fairfax County, Va.

Those who choose to remain are forced to do more with less, working under a far greater, less forgiving microscope, and without many of the past rewards, like unflagging departmental support and family like camaraderie. Many now are so busy doing the job they lose sight of themselves and the impact the work is having on their lives, and relationships, until they are directly asked to reflect, or they are forced to look by circumstances such as when a marriage dissolves, a health crisis occurs or a department complaint is initiated. Then they have no choice, and they are not always happy with the results.

"I've changed. For many years I've been able to separate my job from my personal life. I was able to deal with chaos and not let things get to me emotionally. I am less able to keep my feelings down with calls. The walls are coming down. As of now I'm frequently tearful, even less socialable, and have even more difficulty trusting people. I find it more and more difficult to go to work each day, but I have bills to pay."

Although dispatchers are often identified as the "angry" ones in the public safety family, the professionals most known for their aggression and difficult personality styles, they are not the only ones who are angry.

"I am bitter and snappy at my wife and children. When I stop to think about what happened I get real moody."

John

The first time I met John was during a holiday party for the department. He seemed friendly enough but after only a few minutes of general conversation, the "real" John emerged, or at least the one he had become after "losing" the job he loved. He wasted no time telling me that after 16 years on the job he was angry and bitter about how he'd been demoted and reassigned to "the rubber gun squad" after a chief disagreed with a decision he'd made. Assigned inside to a desk in a division he hated, he counted the days until retirement.

"I have a common cop fantasy now. I want a cabin in the mountains where there are no people. I don't like people anymore. I just want to be alone."

If John only had himself to be concerned with, I suppose living in an isolated cabin high in the mountains wouldn't be much of an issue, if that were his choice. The problem was John wasn't alone. He was married and had been for 6 years. It was his second marriage and her first. Even more problematic then moving off to the wilderness was the fact that his wife, Christine, worked for the department, too, and she enjoyed her job. It was his wife who came into my office seeking help.

Christine

Christine was a tall, attractive woman who dressed well, stayed fit and was roughly 10 years younger than John. They'd met on the job where she worked in the Communications Center. She was far from ready for retirement and still had many plans for herself and her future. Although her current job was adequate, she said, she longed to become a police officer. Since John's demotion, however, his personality had changed dramatically.

"I feel like I'm walking on eggshells all the time. Since my husband's demotion, he's clinically

depressed and angry all the time. I never know what will set him off. I can't talk about anything, and I especially can't talk about anything related to work. I'm afraid one day he'll explode. I don't know if he'll ever get over being demoted, and if he doesn't, I can't live like this."

Look Around You

Many professionals in emergency public safety are stressed.

"I began to think about how my life and attitude had changed since that event and how for two years I couldn't stop thinking about it every day. I would get a sense of dread and not know why. Then it hit me. I was one of several people I had seen a few times throughout my career, a burned out cop... Within two months of finishing the crime scene investigation I had my gall bladder out and was also diagnosed with an ulcer and gerd. Six months after that I was feeling like dirt, sleepy and lethargic and couldn't concentrate. I was sent to a neurologist who in turn sent me to a sleep lab. I was diagnosed as having severe sleep apnea and had surgery for that. I think now that some, if not most of those ailments were in some way caused by stress."

The impact can be enormous, and most times you are not the only one affected.

"I had too high a workload, too few resources and too many areas of responsibility. I withdrew

emotionally from everyone, but my old partner. Eventually this lead to a divorce from my wife."

Deputy Jimmy Hart

"Growing up I heard about officers killing themselves due to the stress of the "job." But I still wanted to do this job as a kid. Once I entered law enforcement I quickly realized that the stress was <u>not</u> from doing your job. The stress came from the administration. Constant Internal Affairs complaints and the threat of losing your job are overwhelming."

Deputy Hart's words were becoming uncomfortably familiar. He'd joined the department because he'd always dreamt of being a cop and now, when he was finally doing the job he'd wanted since he was a small boy growing up on a farm in Indiana, he was desperately afraid of losing it. Why? How could this happen?

I was asked to see this young handsome officer, who took obvious pride in his uniform, because he and his partner had exchanged shots with members of a local gang the night before. Lured into a vehicle pursuit in what turned out to be a highly orchestrated and planned event, the officers responded to a radio broadcast of a 'car jacking' when they were ambushed in an area known for heavy gang affiliation. Snipers shot round after round at the trapped officers with AK47s as they called desperately for backup and returned fire. A heated gun battle ensued until finally backup arrived. In the end, several suspects were arrested. One gang member was shot and killed in the exchange. Miraculously the officers were not wounded.

What startled me most about this particular debriefing was that the officer who sat across from me, who was alive today only by the grace of God, wasn't crying because he was distraught and traumatized by the shooting experience. He was crying because he was consumed by fear about the department's response. Would they blame him? What would the shooting team find on this case? Would the family members of the slain suspect sue him? Would the department back him up, or would it do what it had done in so many other cases, suspend him pending the results of an investigation? Would he lose his job and be unable to support his wife and small child? Would he be disgraced?

Already a veteran of the department's justice system a year earlier, he knew what could happen. During that internal affairs investigation, the fact that the complaint was bogus or his record was spotless was irrelevant; he was treated in "typical" department fashion, "Guilty until proven innocent."

Pending the completion of the Internal Affairs investigation he was assigned to a desk in his division. The investigation took nearly a year to complete during which time other officers shunned him. Supervisors checked up him constantly and without clear reason. Even the Captain took time out to tell him, "I won't put up with officers like you!" In the end, the complaint was unfounded and all charges were dropped. He was returned to patrol like nothing had ever happened, and he was expected to get over it. Now this. Because there was a fatality, and it made the news he expected the worse. He was ready to resign before they fired him and while he could still get another job. He'd been publicly humiliated once. He couldn't put himself or his family through that again.

How had we managed to get to the point where someone who narrowly survived a terrifying near death experience, like an ambush, was more concerned about the possible punitive measures that might be taken by his employer then the sanctity of his own life? Is this what we have come to?

> "As much as I always wanted to do this job, I wish I never did. A businessman could be fired today and working tomorrow. A businessman would not have to discuss why he was fired or the circumstances involved. If a police officer is fired, and it doesn't matter if you are a 30 year veteran or two weeks out of the academy, your law enforcement career is over."

As a psychologist I've listened to many people. Some of the stories I've heard are true and some of the stories I know are far from the truth. I've never seen it as my particular responsibility to investigate the veracity of someone's story. The very fact that someone may come to me and intentionally fabricate a story, for whatever reason, is itself a problem and reason enough to be seen in therapy.

I've also worked in the field long enough to know that some people come in to see therapists just to cover their bases. They're in trouble and if they're asked in court or at a Board of Rights, they want to be able to say that they've been in to see me. They're looking for a reliable witness to support their story. But, I give most people the benefit of the doubt and I try, at a minimum, to be open to their experience of the situation regardless of the facts.

Most people, I do believe, tell me the truth and want help. More times then not, however, I see good men and women who are desperately looking for a way to understand what has happened, and who feel horribly betrayed by an organization they were once willing to give their lives for.

" My police association turned their backs on me. I fought for my job and won. Now everybody's all buddy-buddy again. I haven't forgot."

In the very beginning of my career I'd attributed much of what I'd heard to individual variables. In other words, I believed that what I saw and listened to had more to do with the person and how they lived their lives, then the organization they worked for. If there was a problem or a conflict I looked to see what the person was doing, or not doing, as opposed to necessarily what the organizational system might be creating or perpetuating by it's response or lack thereof. Until I began to notice certain undeniable similarities, and a common theme, if you will, that seemed to predominate certain environments and career fields.

Initially these similarities seemed to exist, and thrive, primarily in dispatch and communications divisions, and certainly many people were more then happy to point the finger there for examples of persistent interpersonal conflicts and overtly angry employees. But, as the public pendulum began swinging in a new less tolerant, even less forgiving direction many department policies and attitudes changed to match. Soon the voices I listened were no longer from Communications Division alone. People were angry, and many with apparent good cause.

How To Tame Your Anger

"Being fired. I wish I could put it behind me and move on. I was eventually re-instated, but to know that my department would fire me over bullshit, and use me to show another department that they won't tolerate an officer like me...it saddens me. I will never forget it."

Clearly, the reasons for the rage we are now seeing in the world and in the workplace are more numerous and complex than maybe even you imagined, but I've tried to give you a short tour of what is out there. Where we go from here is really up to you.

On an organizational level it is unlikely we will see any big changes coming any time soon. Predictions as to when the pendulum will swing back in a favorable direction are extraordinarily difficult to make. The troubles we see are not just one person, or one organization. They are driven by our culture, our society, our organizational systems, our technology and our very way of life.

Before things will change we have to decide that we don't want to live life this way anymore, and that doesn't seem to be the case yet. I'm not sure what will have to happen before enough people decide this is true for them. *In the meantime, what you do have control over is you.*

The following information represents a range of possibilities. Maybe none of them will appeal to you or work for you and the only answer, in your case, is resignation. You may not want to hear this, or want to know this, and in the end you may not even choose it. Despite your anger and unhappiness you may doggedly stay until you reach retirement. I hope, for your sake, that at a minimum you at least attempt to let go of the anger and focus on staying healthy.

Others of you are at least willing to consider the possibilities. This really is your life as you know, and it really is up to you to decide how to live it.

If being in emergency public safety as a cop, or a dispatcher, or an EMT, is that important to you and you're willing to endure the changes regardless of the changing climate, then go for it, but be healthy about it. Some things truly are outside of your hands. Accept it for what it is.

No matter how angry you are with the department or department policy, unless you plan on becoming Chief one day you are unlikely to sway department policy. Influence someone, maybe, impact your supervisors or subordinates by your behavior, also maybe, change public opinion beyond one person at a time, doubtful but affect your own health and well-being and the quality of your life by what decisions you make today, absolutely.

Choose your own life and be accountable for it. You'll be a far happier person for it.

When Confronted With A Situation That Might Trigger An Angry Response:

The following represents *Quick Steps* for managing your anger when confronted by a situation that may trigger it. These are most useful for more immediate needs and are not meant to be the magic pill for more complex situations.

More in-depth methods will be found in Maintaining Morale In The Workplace, and Mindfulness and Stress Management.

Be aware that sometimes the deeper work needs to be done before the simple steps can be taken, but starting some place is better than not starting at all. A stand-alone checklist of Quick Steps will be found in the appendix.

Reason With Yourself

- [ ] **What's really making you angry?**

Usually getting cutoff on the freeway is the just the last straw that breaks the camels back, providing a convenient target for you to unleash your anger about a more difficult issue you may feel unable to resolve, like a failing relationship or the initiation of a complaint against you. Put the anger where it belongs and not on someone or something that isn't even remotely related.

☐ **Is this really important enough to get angry about?**

If you suspend all judgment and just let yourself rip, regardless of the consequences, it's a lot like saying to the universe, "Do with me what you will. I'm yours. I don't care what happens to me or anyone else." Anything can happen, and sometimes it will. Is losing your temper worth everything in your life, as you know it?

☐ **Am I justified in getting angry?**

Sometimes anger is more then justified, but to use an old expression, it's important to "pick your battle." If its that important to you, then by all means go for it and go all the way down to the mat if you need to **but** remember, not everything is worth going down to the mat for, and no matter how angry you are you can still express yourself respectfully, appropriately and with a measure of decorum.

☐ **Will getting angry really make a difference?**

If nothing is to be gained from your anger other than an opportunity to vent, think again. Reconsider your decision. Venting may only fuel the fire and make yourself feel worse.

☐ **Are you feeling early signs of exhaustion or overload?**

While stress alone doesn't cause a blow-up, it makes you more vulnerable to over-reacting. If you're tired or overloaded, take a break, chill out, get some rest, eat some dinner, whatever and then after you're more rested, readdress your initial concerns. If you still have feelings about the person or the situation, then take time to deal with it.

Chill Out

If you're still feeling angry here are some ways to cool off

1. Distract yourself.

2. Breathe

Take slow deep breaths, counting "One" with each successive breath.

3. Withdraw

Sometimes the best solution is to take a time out. Remove yourself from the situation, distance yourself from the person, temporarily, until you have time to cool off, change your perspective, review your frame of reference, think more clearly and rationally.

4. Exercise

Doing physical exercise can be a great release for stress and anger.

5. Laugh at yourself

Not every situation is life or death. Sometimes what we choose to rage about today can seem fairly silly tomorrow, yet at the time we were willing to lose everything over it. Give yourself permission to laugh at yourself, or to change your mind, if you will, at what you are so angry about. Turn arguments into opportunities to laugh with someone else about life's little absurdities and remember what's really important to you both. Most times you'll find its not who forgot to pick up the dry cleaning.

If you're still feeling tempted to let one rip the next time someone cuts you off on the freeway, ask yourself this: **"Why should I let someone I'm never going to see again control my mood and ruin my whole day?"**

THE BEST OF DR 911.COM

Maintaining Morale on the Dispatch Floor

Chapter 3

Maintaining Morale on The Dispatch Floor

The workplace and how you live in it takes more then just showing up everyday. Sometimes it means being brave enough to make the first change: Yourself.

So, is it your responsibility, or my responsibility, or anyone's responsibility for that matter, to see to it that the level of morale within any workplace environment is at a livable level for the individuals who work there? Well, you can probably already guess what I'm going to say. I'm a psychologist. I have a particular bias so OF COURSE you expect me to say something typical like, "I think that there's a relationship between all of the above," and you would be right.

I believe we all have a responsibility towards making the workplace environment one in which people, by and large, feel comfortable, safe, valued and appreciated. It doesn't mean we have to run around the floor doing "touchy-feely" group hugs to the sounds of Kumbaya. In fact, these days if you're not careful doing something like that could set you up for personnel complaint or an order-in visit to the company shrink.

It does mean having a certain level of awareness and, concurrently, having some degree of commitment and felt responsibility towards not only yourself but also towards the work group as a whole.

What You Can't See, Can't Hurt You: WRONG

Dispatcher centers both large and small are microcosms of the larger community. Whether we are referring to the larger community such as the city the center is located in or the organizational community such as the agency that the dispatch center is a part of and works for, the dispatcher who works there is impacted by the community organization. Although separate entities, they are also, in fact, part of a greater whole. One cannot help but be affected by the other and most times what is happening "out there" ultimately influences the mood, temperament and attitude in here and on the floor.

When the larger organization is under fire from the community for whatever the reason, an increase in crime, a sudden surge in community violence resulting in an increase in mortality, a corruption investigation, a use of force investigation, the death of an officer, etc., the smaller organizations within it's umbrella are affected as well.

This may first play out at the command level: as the intensity of the stress organizationally increases (more personnel complaints initiated, uneven promotions, greater accountability on issues that are perceived as unwarranted, reduced perception of "fair and equitable" treatment, etc.), the severity of the stress for the individual intensifies.

It never ever stops where it started.

No one remains untouched: as the command staff feels the pinch the subordinate supervisors are tapped by command to produce. As the pressure heats up on the supervisors, they'll put their subordinates on notice and so forth and so on until it reaches the floor of the dispatch center. In vernacular terms this is a proverbial tale: the man beats the woman who yells at the kid who kicks the dog who chases the cat who pounces on the mouse. Do you get my drift? In the end the mouse has no idea why he was actually pounced on; he just figures it's his due, nor does the cat step back and process why he suddenly decided to pounce on the mouse. He probably thinks it's just because he wanted to and he's a cat, it's his right.

In the land of psychological jargon, we call this a parallel process and this occurs every day whether anyone notices and articulates it or not.

What we mean by this is that if we are not careful or aware we can often times inadvertently emulate many of the same behaviors that our client population exhibits, both good and bad.

Reaching New Thresholds

Example: If I treated only paranoid sex offenders chances are good that after a while, if I'm not careful and I'm not committed to my own healthy well being, my perception of healthy relationships and feeling of safety in the world will become distorted by my persistent exposure to actively paranoid sex offenders.

Even though I am a psychologist I may not actually notice this progressive distortion of my reality, "Can't see the forest for the trees." But realistically and also depending on my individual personality characteristics *after time my basic threshold for tolerating bizarre distorted behavior will shift and a new baseline will become established.*

Someone from the outside, like family, might see this change and say, "Whoa! What's going on here?" but someone on the inside, such as another colleague doing the same kind of work, may not even notice, and in fact, may inadvertently reinforce this transformation *because it is also happening within themselves.*

Translating this into law enforcement: As individuals starting our careers in law enforcement we may have been easy going, tolerant, innocent, friendly, and open minded. But as the sands of times shift down, after a number of years on the job we may find that we have become critical, judgmental, opinionated, "paranoid," concrete and aggressive.

Sometimes we are the ones who notice this change in ourselves but frequently it is a family member or friend who points this out to us. If it is on the job, it will often times be identified, as **"that's just the way it is here."**

Is this just an expected by-product of the job? Maybe, but it doesn't necessarily always have to be this way unless you decide you want it to be this way. For example, one would not be expected to suspend judgment when rolling out to a" hot prowl" or responding to an "officer needs help" call. *But if you're not handling a call and yet you're treating your co-workers the same way you treat a suspect or a PR, then Houston, we have a problem.*

But, you say, "Just because you're paranoid doesn't mean someone's not out to get you." True, but there's a limit to what is appropriate and manageable behavior.

I worked for a large organization that these days seems to be hip deep in problems, complaints and litigation. It's hard to pick up the newspaper without reading something about the department.

Does this have an impact on the people who work hard everyday doing the best job they know how to even when they have little or nothing to do with the events they hear about on the news?

Absolutely, because ultimately the stress of the organization filters through to the people on the floor. When, where and how it affects you may simply depend on where you are on the "food chain," but ultimately you will be affected.

This can be experienced as helplessness, hopelessness, depression, anger, demoralization or apathy. It can mean different things to different people, but like the elephant in the room, just cause you don't talk about it doesn't mean that it isn't there.

The bottom line is we all bear some responsibility towards maintaining the morale level of the organization, both individually for ourselves as human beings, but also as colleagues, supervisors, peers, team members, instructors, friends and subordinates.

At times, within any organization, people aren't always fair or sensitive, but that's just part of life.

Unfortunately, it seems that the more successful or content you may feel in your life the more likely people may try to cut you down. Either way you slice it, no matter what the story is, fair or unfair, you have to help you, and in doing so, ultimately you help the organization.

When Personal and Professional Lives Collide

For years I was angry. The life I'd been dealt wasn't the one I asked for or expected. True, when it all began I wasn't old enough to know the difference, nor could I have changed the course of events even if I'd wanted to, but as an adult I was forced to live with the outcome. This wasn't the plan. *Didn't anyone know that yet? What did I have to do to get somebody's attention?*

With one single event my entire life changed. Everything I thought I knew was certain was replaced by people and places I'd never known before, and didn't particularly want to know now. No one asked me if this is what I wanted, but then at 14, who does? I didn't understand what was happening and no one seemed to want to be the one to tell me.

Before my mother died I believe she did everything she knew how to do to try and create some sort of life for her children after she was gone. Startling naïve, and sadly alone in her endeavors, she tried to set everything up as best she could with her own limited resources, hoping that it would be enough for us to survive, but in the end things happened so quickly. In one short year she was gone, and once she passed, it was all out of her hands.

30 years later I've learned that in life much of what happens is out of our control. I only wish that it hadn't taken me so long to learn it. Had my mother lived instead of dying at the age of 46, my age now, I can't imagine she would have intended on the troubled times her children endured. I think she probably expected that people would do the right thing, and seeing the situation we were in, would rise to the occasion and pitch in, come to our rescue, and help us but few people ever did.

This doesn't mean that people weren't kind to us, if the "right" situation presented itself, but it takes more then simple moments of kindness to put food on the table or clothing on children's backs.

Same As It Ever Was

I've spent most of my adult life trying to unlearn what was so indelibly imprinted on my brain and in my heart as a young woman growing up in an unpredictable world without parents: that the world is an unsafe place, that people can't be trusted, that the only person you can really trust is yourself, and that if given half a chance most people will take advantage of you, and use and abuse you, especially if you're a child. I had a lot to be angry about.

When people told me things like, "You have to learn to love yourself before you can love other people," I looked at them like they had two heads and no brain between them. My face may have been smiling, but my heart was saying 'You're nuts!' I knew what people were capable of. I'd been there and done that and I believed these words like I believed I really could buy the Brooklyn Bridge. *"You don't know what it's really like to be here, to be me."*

If you'd asked me back then I couldn't have told you what I was so angry about. I didn't know. I didn't even know I was angry. This was just my life as I had come to know it. It never occurred to me that it could be any other way.

No matter how hurt I felt by something or someone I never said anything. How could I? I couldn't risk even the smallest infraction or deviation from the norm. No chance to be rejected. I needed food. I needed shelter. I needed someone to care. Every part of me screamed, "love me!" but every gesture, nuance and outward behavior insisted that I wanted distance and detachment. I was independent and no one would ever hurt me like I'd been hurt before. Years had to pass, along with several bad relationships, and a series of wildly different careers, before I finally stopped long enough to see the impact my life had on me.

At first I didn't want to look. I didn't want to know. I just wanted things to be better. But I didn't really want to change anything, or do anything myself to make it better.

I told myself that *anyone who knew me should know what I wanted*, simply by being around me. "I shouldn't have to tell them" I said, but secretly I was too afraid to ask. What if they said, "No"? Every time someone stepped all over me, because he or she didn't have a clue what I wanted, since I'd never told anyone to begin with, I was devastated but I still didn't change anything. I didn't know how. Life seemed to be one big mystery to me, except for the pain, that was familiar.

In my early twenties I told a friend, "I want there to be a book, a Dell paperback, that I can buy for 99 cents at the supermarket and in this book I want it to tell me everything I should do in my life, and I would do it and it would be right."

I never found that book.

I was prey in a world of predators, and like any young woman growing up unprotected by normal constraints can tell you, life was hard. But I didn't understand what all this meant, or how my life had changed as a consequence of these experiences until I reached graduate school.

Once More, With Feeling

Graduate school for psychologists is a lot like being in therapy all of the time, 24/7/365 days a year. Students live, breathe and eat psychology and everything you feel, think and experience is examined, reexamined and then discussed in minute detail, and then just when you think you've discussed it enough, you look at it again.

The goal is the development of awareness. The process isn't the same for everyone nor does life suddenly become easier or necessarily "instantly better" because you have insight into your own behavior but it's a step in the right direction, or so they say.

Blindness is bliss. If the only feelings you pay attention to are your own, and only in service to your own ego gratification, then how great is that? No responsibilities for anyone else's feelings. No worries. No need to care about anyone else other then yourself. Cool, but unless you really are the true definition of a narcissist, it isn't any happier. Most people want to care for someone in their lives, and in turn want to be cared for. The challenge is that a relationship is always easier until we add another person to it.

Awareness is a double-edged sword. Choosing awareness is choosing to see; it's choosing to be honest with your self deep in your heart of hearts; it's choosing to operate with integrity. You are your word. As much as it means the potential for happiness, it also means that sometimes you are in the position of making the hard decision.

You may be the only one in the room, or the relationship, who really sees what's going on. The burden of responsibility falls to you and that's the biggest challenge. Do you rise to the occasion, or do you keep your mouth shut, not say anything and hope that it works out?

It's a tough call to make. It's especially tough in the beginning, when you are still learning. *Decisions don't become easier as we become more practiced but we spend less time in pain over the outcome. We learn to take responsibility for what we can and let the rest go.*

Clients often complain that they had more fun before they were aware of what they were doing.

"Before I started therapy I could go out with someone, have sex and it was no big deal. Didn't matter that she wanted a relationship with me. I was honest. I told her I wasn't interested. If she wanted to fool around, great, if she didn't, that was ok too, there were plenty more where she came from. She always said yes, but then after we went out a few times we'd always end up arguing. I never said I'd date only her and then when I did exactly what I said I was going to do, she'd get mad! She never believed me. Now, I understand what I was doing, and I can't do it anymore! This is no fun!"

Like my client, once he saw that his actions were hurting his girlfriend, he couldn't not take responsibility for the pain he was inflicting. He was accountable for his actions. He had a choice to make.

Once you cross that invisible line into awareness, its harder and harder not to see how everything we do, and don't do, has an impact in the world.

In my office I've often found that the person with the greater awareness is usually the one who identifies herself as the problem. Many times I hear,

" I'm the only one who seems to have a problem with this. My boyfriend tells me I'm too sensitive. So what if he looks at pornography all the time, leaves it out for the kids to see and goes to strip joints every chance he can get. He's just having fun. It doesn't mean anything. My friends tell me to get over it, and stop having so many feelings about it. It's no big deal, but I don't like it. It doesn't make me feel good, so I thought I'd come into therapy so that I can learn how not to have feelings anymore. OK?"

But living a happier life isn't about getting better at not feeling, or caring, anymore. It's about getting better and better about knowing how you really feel. No lies, no pretenses, no omissions of truth or subtleties of misinformation, and then doing something about it. Acting on your feelings.

After death many people respond to loss with denial. The first few years after my mother died I kept waiting for her home to come home. Of course I knew she had died and that wasn't possible, but emotionally I was still in denial. It was as though she'd gone to the store and any minute now she'd come home and everything would be back to normal and we would be ok again. When that didn't happen, and time began to stretch out behind me like an empty highway that no one traveled on anymore, a feeling of longing for her, or someone like her, began pervading every part of my life, everything I did and everyone I came into contact with.

Automatic Pilot

Looking back I'm reminded of when I install a new program on my computers hard drive. After the systems program is installed a little icon pops up on the bottom of the screen to let me know that while I'm doing other kinds of work, the program I've installed is silently running in the background. I don't need to select the icon for the program to work. It's always running in the background, waiting for the right data to present itself to begin the process. I don't even have to think about it because it is programmed into the system. It functions whether I am aware of it or not.

Early experiences in life are a lot like this computer program. They hardwire us to respond in a certain way to life experiences, and like the computer program, they're always running in the background. Day after day, from one minute to the next, at work and at home, the program is running but our immediate level of awareness varies. We may be reminded by specific events that occurred that are obvious to us, a birthday, a death or an anniversary, but mostly we don't even notice the program's running.

Unless we delete it from the hard drive or learn how to modify the programs contents, which takes more sophisticated knowledge or technical expertise, the program merrily runs in the background, regardless of what we are doing, silently gathering information from our experiences, and waiting for that opportunity to open.

At times within any system people aren't always fair or sensitive, but that's part of life. I didn't ask for the life I had as a child, or for my mother to die, but that's what happened. I can either spend the rest of my life mired in my own despair, depression, disappointment or anger and resentment, or move on. I can either pick people who will continue to reinforce the belief that the world is an unsafe place and no one can be trusted, or I can move on and learn to pick differently.

This is always my choice.

I may not want to hear this. I may not want to see this. I may not want to admit this, but the bottom line is: It is always my choice. It has always been my choice. It will always be my choice. I may not be able to choose the circumstances, but I can always choose my response to it.

Unfortunately, it seems that the happier and more successful you are, the more other people look at this as an opportunity to cut you down, but so be it. No matter what the story is, good or bad, fair or unfair, you have to be willing to help you. In doing so, ultimately everyone benefits.

You Create Your Own Experience

Organizations, corporations, family systems, relationships, friendships all contain within themselves their own "life" force or energy. Given enough momentum by the people operating within the system and any situation can take on a "life of its own."

We've all been the targets of that force at one time or another in our lives. At the best of times we feel embraced and supported. Warm in the arms of our "family" we are content to remain in the safety of its "love." It feels too good to leave.

At the worst of times we feel attacked, undermined and misunderstood. Bereft with loss, when the family rejects or abandons us, we feel humiliated and betrayed.

Despite your beliefs about the system or your role in it, you have everything to do with what your life experiences are when you are there.

You are accountable for your life. Whether you are on the job or at home, at a crime scene or in the car, in uniform or plain clothes, retired or getting ready to do so, good, bad or indifferent, happy or sad, fair or unfair, no matter where you are, you own your own life. Acknowledge and accept responsibility for this. Understand your role in creating the results that are your life, both on the job and at home. You may think that relationships just happen, or that people are doing something to you, but they don't. You have something to do with how you experience what you see and feel. Learn to choose better so you have better.

You have always been accountable. You will always be accountable. That's how it is. You may not like it. You may want to resist it. This may not be how you would like it to be, but that's how it is. If you don't like your job, you are accountable. If you're having trouble with your marriage, you are accountable. If you're having conflicts with coworkers on the job, you are accountable. If you are depressed, angry, sad, glad, you are accountable.

Whatever circumstances we are talking about, the reality is you have something to do with how you experience it. This means, if you're willing to accept this belief, that you can no longer **"not see."** You can't dodge the responsibility for what is your life.

This doesn't mean just saying the words, or acting politically correct, or saying one thing and doing another. This means living your life being responsible for the outcome of your experiences, and how you contribute this experience to whatever system you are a part of.

If we're talking about work and your relationship with your supervisor is bad, you had something to do with creating that "bad" relationship. If you choose not to see this, then every decision you make from this point on is influenced by this distortion in perception. Even if you think that there can't possibly be a link between the chaos at work and yourself, think again.

You have something, everything and nothing to do with what is going on in your life. You may really believe that its out of your hands but the fact is, if you're miserable at work, you have everything to do with maintaining that misery, but you have to chose to see it before you can change it. If you truly want to change, if you truly want things to be better at work with your boss, or at home in your relationship, then you need to get abundantly clear with yourself about who is accountable for what you see.

You must carefully look at what you've done or haven't done to create the undesirable results. *"Well, I haven't done anything. It just happened!"* Nothing just happens. Look again.

This isn't about attributing blame or getting better at pointing the finger at someone else. This is simply about seeing what part you have in perpetuating and stopping an undesirable or unwanted behavior or experience.

You Can Not Change What You Can Not See

For so much of what we do in life we're on automatic pilot. Life becomes routine. Even the tasks we enjoy we lose our sense of pleasure from as they are seamlessly interwoven with the rest of our lives. In service to our needs to get the job done, we forget to feel anything while we're doing it.

Arriving at home after a long day on the job, we have no memory of the drive or what we thought about. Having Friday night sex with our partner, we review the shopping list in our minds or tally up the bills we need to pay. Taking a report from a tearful victim, we think about tee off time at the course and whether we brought the extra pair of socks. Waking up with a knot in your stomach and a sour taste in your mouth, you get ready for work like an automaton, feeling nothing, seeing nothing, just putting the clothes on, one foot in front of the other.

A means to an end, the day is only worth waking up to because you know at 1530, you're one day closer to retirement.

What you are doing or not doing is a choice. It may not feel like a choice to you at this moment but it is. This is your life. If you project responsibility for everything that happens to you onto everyone else, "bad instructors," "bad supervisors," "unfair rules," "hostile work environment," "crazy people," then you abdicate responsibility and control over what happens next in your life.

If morale on the job is at it lowest point in a decade and you turn away because you believe it's not your responsibility to change things for someone else then why should it surprise you when nothing changes and the bad situation continues?

If you haven't spent more then two minutes with your kids except for when you were yelling at them for what they haven't done right then why should it surprise you when their grades start slipping or they act like they can't hear you?

If you haven't told your wife you loved her or held her close simply for the sake holding her, because she means something of value to you, since the last time you wanted sex, then why should you be surprised when she loses interest in being sexually intimate with you?

Get real with yourself about your life and everybody in it. Be truthful about what isn't working in your life both on the job and at home. Stop making excuses and start making results. You can do this.

Being honest with yourself means taking responsibility for what you see, and taking responsibility for what you see means doing something to change it. You could wait for someone else to come along to do it for you but chances are you could wait for a very long time, or you could wait until something occurs that forces some kind of change for you, but you may not be very happy with the results. It could be worse then what you started with. You could wait until someone else "gets it" and understands how unhappy or angry you are with them, but even if they get it they're under no obligation to do anything to change your life. It's just not their responsibility. It's yours.

When the retaliation started I was heart broken. For months I had agonized over the situation at work, talking to everyone under the sun in my personal life about the problems I was having on the job with a co-worker and with the work group I was part of. No matter how much his behavior bothered me, I was more afraid of what could happen if I said anything to anyone in the office then I was of tolerating the discomfort.

Despite working in a high profile highly specialized career field, the dominant culture within the office was no different then others I heard about from my clients.

On more then one occasion I'd witnessed the public humiliation and devaluing of female professional staff who dared to disagree with group consensus and make their opinion public. Speak up too many times and you risked being shunned and ostracized by your peers.

The "boss" did nothing to stem the tide. If I said anything I would be out there on my own and from that point on anything could happen. Based on what I listened to in my office from people on the job, it usually did.

I needed my job. Whereas others on the department could transfer to another section, there were few, if any places, we could go, except resignation. I wasn't ready to resign, but I wasn't ready to say anything yet.

Years of living at below the poverty level after my mother died left me with an indelible impression. I never wanted to be hungry and homeless again.

As irrational as I knew this fear was it still preyed on me. What if I couldn't find another job? "I will never be without a job again," I would tell myself. "There's always McDonalds. Worse case scenario I'll flip hamburgers for a living until I find something." But even that didn't convince me I'd be OK.

Of equal, if not greater concern, was my fear of retaliation by my colleagues. What would they do? Assuming they would do nothing because we were a group of highly educated professionals was unrealistic at best given what I'd been witness to, but would they really turn against me as I feared?

Talking to anyone outside of the section is breaking the cardinal rule, and keeping "the secret" is the first priority in abusive dysfunctional families. Only the abusers are allowed to make up the rules, everyone else is expected to go along with the program or risk their own destruction. Our group was no different.

I'd spent years learning how to "pass." Kids without parents or adult guardians grow up learning how to find their way in an increasingly hostile world, one that is always looking to take advantage of your vulnerabilities. While our culture has more systems in place now to take care of children, and protect their rights, and their bodies, child abuse still occurs with painful regularity.

In my time, there was little protection afforded by social services and most "good" adults were afraid to "get involved." No one wanted to take responsibility for helping out because what if something went wrong? They might get blamed and then where they would be? Up a creek without a paddle so most times "good" adults just watched on the sidelines.

The "bad" people, the abusers, the molesters, and other people you most wanted to keep your children away from, were always first in line to help out whenever they could. They looked great on the outside, but once you walked through the door they opened, it slammed behind you, and hit you on the butt going in. If you were lucky you could get it back open again and get out. But if you weren't, then that's where you stayed until whoever was keeping you there got tired of you. Who knew how long that would be?

I was a bright kid. It didn't take me long to realize that if I planned on living through my childhood I'd need to get street smart in a heart beat, or I'd end up dead, in jail or living out my life in a minimum wage job on the island with a brood of kids of my own.

My number one survival tactic was learning how to "pass," or fit in with whatever group I was surrounded by. Blending in with the scenery I tried not to take up too much space or bring too much attention to myself personally. Other people generally felt free to do and be and say whatever they wanted to around me, but I never really said much about myself. It was the safest bet towards survival, my own.

Humpty Dumpty Sat On A Wall…

My fears kept me silent, but in the end my silence nearly destroyed me. When my worst fears were realized after I spoke out, and my colleagues acted out against me in exactly the way I predicted I wanted to blame them for hurting me. I wanted to blame the department for not acting on my concerns when I first reported them. I wanted to blame my boss for lacking the skills needed to create a safe work environment, free of sexual innuendo, overt hostility and discriminatory practices. I wanted to blame those who encouraged me to report for not protecting me or supporting me through the process like they promised.

But, if I am really honest with myself none of that excused me from looking at the part I played in creating the situation, and I did have something to do with what occurred.

I was upset and I was angry, but I hadn't really wanted to do anything. On the basis of who I was alone, I believed I'd already endured enough. I thought people knew me. I thought it was someone else's turn to come in, and take responsibility for making the wrongs right.

Why was it my responsibility to "bell the cat?"

So, after I made the initial reports I said nothing, and after the retaliation began, first in small childish ways and then building into directed hostility, slanderous statements and outright misconduct, I endured. I did my work. I smiled. I would not allow myself to act in the same ways towards others that they did towards me.

I waited for "justice" to be done, for those in positions of power to "get it," to finally understand the importance of what I was talking about: that people who are tasked with the responsibility of providing mental health services should be the first to live their lives above reproach, and that as psychologists it was not only our moral and ethical obligation to do so as clinicians, but also as human beings who were part of the greater universe. We of all people should be willing to walk what we talked.

We should be more willing to police our own behavior and own what belonged to us than the "average Joe." We should be first to eliminate "bad" behavior, or behavior that is intentionally misguided, cruel, devaluing and destructive, and if we engaged in inappropriate behavior even if unintentionally, then we should be committed to looking at what point we failed. We shouldn't have to be told this, or so I thought.

"We should be the safest place in the department," I would say to anyone who listened, "but we're not. Why doesn't anyone get that?" Nothing changed.

I kept telling myself that it would get better, but everyday it seemed to get worse. When clients sat in my office talking about their own experiences on the job, I sat there silent about my own. Certainly it wasn't my place to talk about myself with my clients, but inside, as I listened to their pain, I felt my own throb with intensity.

At what point would I change? When would I decide that enough was enough? My health had already started deteriorating when the stress intensified to extraordinary levels. Would I wait until a life-threatening crisis occurred and that would signal, "Enough"?

The Point of Reckoning

Had I valued myself, and my own self worth, for more then just as a vehicle for helping others with their pain and unhappiness, then the very second the red flag was on the horizon, at the first sighting of inappropriate behavior or misconduct of any kind, it was my responsibility to say something, or do something, to set things right, even if it meant walking out of there.

Had I taken responsibility and held myself accountable for my own life, I would never have found myself in a situation that nearly destroyed everything about myself that I valued. But from the very first moment I stepped into the office, while sitting in the front room waiting for my first interview to the actual interview itself, I knew something was wrong. The intuitive voices were blasting inside my head but I didn't want to hear what they were saying because to hear them meant **change**.

I didn't want to change. I wanted a job. I wanted to come back to California. I wanted to be near things that I remembered and people who were familiar to me. This was my vehicle for returning, for answering my dreams, and wasn't it my turn to dream?

If I chose to see what was really in front of me, that there was something deeply wrong and dysfunctional within the system I would become a part of, then I would have had to say no to my dream of the future. So, I chose not to see, and like that computer program silently running in the background, I knew that accepting this job carried with it the potential for placing myself in harms way. But, I didn't want to see this.

Whatever I was feeling and seeing on that first day was silently running in the background, collecting data and waiting for the opportunity to open and take over. In that moment I said to the universe, "Do with me what you will. My life is yours for the asking," and I set a ball into motion that would take years before it stopped rolling.

Despite all my years of education and training, all my experiences as an independent successful professional, all the challenges I endured and overcame in childhood, there are some moments in time that happen that could be summed up into three words, "She forgot everything." I may be the person that people paid money to talk to, who was supposed to know things, an "expert", but in some situations I am a vulnerable human being in an enormous universe just trying to find my way home.

The lessons I learned in childhood were some of the most powerful lessons I had learned in my life. Although I knew I would never go hungry again, or be forced to do something I would later feel ashamed of, because I needed to survive, somewhere deep in my heart there remained a memory that I wasn't worth fighting for. I was embarrassed, and ashamed, that someone of my age, training, and experience was in a situation that I found to be profoundly humiliating. What would my clients and my colleagues outside of the department think if they knew? By judging myself, and then by not accepting accountability for my part in what was happening, I allowed myself to, once again, become prey in a world of predators.

Get real with yourself about your life and everybody in it. Be truthful about what isn't working in your life, both at home and on the job. Stop making excuses and start making results.

Being honest with yourself means taking responsibility for what you see, and taking responsibility for what you see means doing something to change it.

You could wait for someone else to come along to do it for you but chances are you could wait a very long time. If you're unwilling to acknowledge a thought, circumstance, problem, condition, feeling or behavior, if you won't take ownership of your role in the situation then you cannot and will not change it.

If you refuse to acknowledge your own self destructive tendencies, on the job or off, then not only will they continue they will actually gain power and momentum, become more deeply entrenched in the habitual patterns of your life, more deeply engrained in the operating systems of your department, and grow more and more resistant to change.

One of my colleagues on the job confided,

"Until you said something I'd stop noticing how bad it really was. I used to eat my lunch in my car because it was so bad in the office. I couldn't be there unless I absolutely had to, but I just got used to it. Nothing ever seemed to change, so I just stopped trying."

Walking a tightrope between what you can endure on the job in exchange for what you can get out of the job, (special off duty jobs, "self-respect" off the job, good pay, more attention from women) is a precarious venture. You may be able to keep the job, but lose yourself in the process.

Denial is a functional defense, and it is also the number one obstacle to change. You cannot change what you cannot, or will not, see. No matter how bad it is it's never too late to do something. But be honest about what needs to be done.

There are many meaningful aspects of who you are and what you create in your life. You may have chosen to accommodate or incorporate these aspects and characteristics into your life. If you ignore or deny the fact that these characteristics in you have influenced how you interact with others, then you are denying an important aspect of your life.

When it came to my clients I was always willing to go down to the mat for them. Fighting for the rights of someone else and their livelihood was a battle I would take on without a moment's hesitation.

Defending a theoretical concept, challenging an entrenched systemic organizational belief, protesting an endangered species or way of life, were the bread and butter of my job, and my life, and I relished the opportunities to prove my mettle. Advocating for a downtrodden group or protecting the rights of other women and children, family members, animals were right up my alley and I advocated tirelessly without any hesitation or felt anxiety.

But, when it came to me and the moment I was attacked personally and on a very primitive level, behavior that was sexually motivated and driven by a male colleague, I folded.

Had there been just one person within my own department who demonstrated the kind of fearless support I needed, who wasn't also motivated by protecting their own needs in a dangerous environment, maybe the path I would have traveled on would have been less painful, less circuitous then the one I took. But only parents, if you're lucky, and people like Mother Teresa and Gandhi, are that selfless, so to expect that from anyone was unrealistic.

It was always my responsibility to take care of me, and so in denying my own feelings about what I saw, and the people in my life, I became part of the problem.

In my silence I became complicit to the persistent distortions of the truth that existed within my section. The more I chose to endure, the more power I gave away. Articulating their own anger, frustration and fears, my clients served as a daily reminder of my shame. When it came to my own needs I was a person and not a professional. My silence gave them power.

If you do not acknowledge the presence of the distorting characteristic or event, whatever that is, and you do not acknowledge that you really own it or have a part in it, then you cannot or will not ever escape that experience.

You might change jobs, or change relationships, but you will not change the eventuality of that experience.

Owning your own experience doesn't mean projecting blame, or becoming a professional victim, "Everything's my fault because I'm not smart enough." You're just letting yourself off the hook if you buy into that, and if change is what you want then you need to stay on that hook. The discomfort you are feeling is a red flag you need to see.

Acknowledge for real that you can make choices for change. Effecting meaningful and lasting change in your life is difficult enough even under the best of circumstances. Don't make it worse by making assumptions or by being naïve about what's really happening around you. Don't be fooled by your own self-talk, anymore then you would allow yourself to be fooled by a suspect, or one of your kids.

If you're going to make a difference in your life, whether on the job or at home, then you have to be honest with yourself. Time to start opening your eyes.

I told myself that those tasked with the responsibility of helping me were doing so because they were motivated by their own integrity and the need to do what is right. Even when their behavior at times seemed suspect, and their motivations seemed more driven by political aspirations then their concern for me, I convinced myself I was wrong. I believed that in the end, everyone, including the department, would do the "right thing." It wasn't until the final straw that broke the camels back, that I opened my eyes and realized that individuals may care about me, but the organization only "cared" about the organization. I was expendable. It wasn't personal.

As long as the department took enough steps to demonstrate "something" was done in response to the problem, then in the eyes of all those who looked that was enough. If that wasn't enough for me, then I'd better open my eyes and start being more honest with myself about what I wanted, and on what I was willing to do to get it.

You get back what you put into it.

Sometimes it seems that the one activity people have more time for then any other activity is talking about other people, downing a person, or a place, or a situation. "Negative Thoughts-R-Us," predominates the work environment as though it's the only language some people know. To say something nice about someone else would kill them.

The work or home environment only has to remain a negative one if you agree to keep it that way, either by your denial of its existence, your resistance to doing something about it, or your own active participation in creating and perpetuating it.

But if you what you want is to be treated well and with respect, fairly and with integrity then start by treating others with respect, fairly and with integrity. "Treat others as you would wish to be treated" isn't just an old saying. Live what you believe. If you believe in good things happening to good people, that generating positive energy is a worthwhile expression of energy and that it's important to treat all people with a measure of kindness and respect, then live your life that way no matter where you are. Not just at home and not in the field or in the division.

Even a colleague who stands accused in a disciplinary action or a suspect you've just arrested deserves to be treated with kindness, respect and integrity. Every opportunity in life is a chance to make a choice, to practice kindness in every interaction no matter where you are or who you are with.

People only do what works. Regardless of what somebody may tell you, or what you may be telling yourself, if someone is knowingly engaged in negative and destructive behavior, and he or she does it anyway, they are getting something out of it. In some way it works for them.

I ask clients all the time, "What are you getting out of staying in that destructive relationship? You're miserable. He's abusive to you. What do you get out it?" 9 out of 10 times they tell me, "Nothing." Wrong.

If you're staying you're getting something from the process. It's not a good thing, or a life affirming life-enhancing thing, but you are getting something.

When we're talking about an abusivc relationship, it might be that you believe in your heart this is the only kind of relationship you can have, or that you deserve. *If people really knew you then they would know how unlovable you really are and in the end they would leave you anyway.* So, you stay because you don't believe it could be any other way. You'll never be treated any better or differently.

People also stay hooked into a negative experience if they're getting some kind of payoff, or if they are expecting some kind of payoff, in the end. Until they're willing to risk giving that something up, I mean really give it up, they will resist change. In fact, they will hold onto it for dear life even if the effects are killing them, ruining their relationship, wreaking havoc on their health or destroying their credibility on the job. They're not letting go.

In the workplace this translates into perceived power. "What power," you may ask. "We're all in the same boat here." Well, it may be power over who counts the paperclips but its perceived as power nonetheless, and some people will fight tooth and nail to keep it or have some part in deciding who has a right to count the paperclips.

Working in an environment that consisted of "all chiefs and no Indians," as I did, power and who had it was an enormous concern and focus of energy for those I worked with. Although those on the outside would expect an office of mental health professionals to be at a minimum warm, supportive, respectful and open, our office rarely met those expectations. Superficially we gave the appearance of doing the right thing, we were bright enough not to risk poisoning the cow we got the milk from, but behind the scenes the battle roared. Lines were drawn around gender, money, intellectual prowess, age, sexual attractiveness, and almost any situation that provided someone an opportunity to take a step up on the back of someone else.

In Southern California, the land of the beautiful, there were many opportunities and this particular type of social currency counted for a lot.

Sometimes what people are getting from the experience is not always obvious to you, or me, or even the person who is doing the battling. He or she may persist in being negative at work, towards anyone who will listen, because deep in their heart and minds is a belief that they don't deserve any better. So, even if they complain about the job, they won't do anything to change it. It may not make sense to you, but it doesn't have to make sense to you to change it.

Identify the payoffs that are driving the behavior and you have a chance at changing the behavior. If you want it all, then you have to be willing to risk it all, and that means giving up negative concepts about yourself and others.

I needed to acknowledge that pursuing the course I was on would ultimately lead to my own destruction. It had already come at great cost to me. If I remained it could be my life. If I wanted to get the life I deserved then I had to be willing to risk everything.

I had to acknowledge that regardless of what I wanted for my work group, or for the people I treated or did consultations with, as long as nothing else changed in my work environment, as long as the key players remained the same and the department remained entrenched in their own familiar organizational practices, undisputed, my life in the department would not change. Things would never be made right. It would be better for those who came after me, but it would never be for me in the way that was important to me.

No one could put the genie back in the bottle again. I may have wanted to move on, but others were not about to let me. They wanted me to pay.

Become one of the people who get it. The world is filled with people who don't get it. This seems like such a simple fundamental concept that its funny to say it but having been there and done that, it's a critically important one and needs to be identified.

Look around you. In almost every situation there are people who get it, and people who don't get it, and it is really easy to tell them apart. You know it. You see it every day. There are the people who work hard every day and have a good time doing it, no matter what they do or where they are, and they're not afraid to show it. Then, there are the people who don't get it. Who spend more time then not, beating their head against the walls a few hundred times, complaining about everyone, how unfair life is and how they can never seem to get a break.

Those who get it seem to go with the flow. They're not arrogant, or pretentious, or obnoxiously self centered. They just don't spend a whole lot of time in counterproductive behavior. If it doesn't work, they move on and let it go. They're successful at home and at work because they've acquired the knowledge they need to create the results they want.

Knowing how to be an effective manager of others is helpful, it is exponentially more important to be an effective manager of your self.

No matter where you are or what the circumstances are where you encounter people, the one common denominator is you. You are the one person you spend the most time with. You are only person you know with absolute certainty you will spend the rest of your life with. More then anyone else on the job, at home, or at the Laundromat, the one person you most need the power to influence and control is you.

The person whose negative characteristics and behavior patterns you most need to manage or eliminate, and whose positive life affirming life supporting behavior you most need to maximize is you. Whether the characteristic is anger, depression, sadness, aggression, apathy, insecurity, despair, or any other of a number of possible characteristics, you are the one who will have to minimize or eliminate it. Doing so requires time, knowledge and patience. It takes knowledge about how you developed that negative characteristic, why you persist in having it, and more importantly how to replace it with more positive constructive characteristics.

So as much as knowledge and information are power, the lack of knowledge or the reliancc on distorted information is misleading, destructive and harmful. Decide now that you will gather knowledge about how and why you and those you encounter in life do what you, and they, do. Let this inform you as to what becomes the bedrock of the knowledge you will learn to draw from. Listen to the voices within you. They are trying to be heard.

There is Power in Forgiveness

Many times on the job I've heard that people have long memories. **"It may have been 10 years ago that I made that mistake, but around here people act like it was yesterday."**

Open your eyes to what anger and resentment are doing to you. Take your power back from those who have hurt you.

Of all the emotions in our vast range of human experiences, anger, hate and resentment are amongst the most powerful and the most destructive. They come alive within you by the actions of those who you perceive to have hurt you or those you love.

You may think that you are justified in how you feel or what you do. You may truly believe that your anger or rage is what you want and need to handle a situation because someone has hurt you deeply enough to create these emotions. You may believe that they deserve it and are made to suffer by your hatred of them. You may sometimes treat your anger and hatred as though it has its' own life force, and is something outside of yourself that you have no control over. But to do so, to carry this hatred around with you, and to feel this hatred within you is to pay an unbelievable high price, for the everyday reality of these feelings change the very core of who you are. They change your heart, they change your mind and if you have a spiritual belief, they change your soul.

These feelings can become so pervasive that they can crowd out every other kind of feeling that exists for you, consuming you with behavior that is vicious, manipulative, aggressive, antagonistic, bitter, internally and externally, at home and at work.

Think about it. When you encounter someone like that at work who's in the grip of these emotions, it rolls off them in giant waves of emotion. You can feel the negative energy that emanates from them and it takes little imagination to guess what must be going on inside. Hatred, anger, and resentment eat away at the very fabric of ones heart and soul.

Are you really going to be the caretaker of that hatred, anger and resentment for the rest of your life? Do you really believe that you can keep these feelings only at work, that they don't permeate and become a part of every part of your existence no matter where you are?

Don't do it another day. You have the power to forgive these people—not as a gift to them, but as a gift to yourself. You are worth whatever it takes to rise above the hurt, the pain, and the grief. But remember you create your own experience. You have the resolve to create what you want, and rid yourself of what you don't want. If that person benefits from your forgiveness, then so be it. The person you are out to save is you. The one who's being held an emotional hostage is you.

The power of forgiveness is the power to set yourself free from the bonds of anger, hatred, and resentment. Seize the moment and rise above. You are worth it, and everyone you know and love deserves it.

Taking Your First Steps Towards Healing

Chapter 4

Creating Health

FOR HELPING PROFESSIONALS

In life there are an infinite range of choices open and available to each and every one of us, every day and in every moment. Yet, despite this poor health, destructive relationships, and negative work environments often challenge our lives and pervade every aspect of it. We feel helpless to change and yet know that change is crucial to our happiness.

For those of us in helping professions, this dichotomy is a double-edged sword and a source of guilt and shame. We, who are tasked with helping others to sort out and survive their lives, are often unable to do the same for ourselves in our own lives.

How To Make Sense Out of This?

I'll never forget the conversation I had with a young female police officer who was herself the victim of severe domestic abuse.

Officer Janet Page

For years Officer Page lived with a brutal man who routinely beat her and with whom she stayed yet steadfastly refused to leave. As is the frequent case for many women (and men) who are in this position, she made excuses for his behavior and continued to believe and hope that the rare glimpses she had of the man she once knew signified a return to the man he was when they'd married.

As a patrol officer she routinely responded to domestic calls with her partner, who was unaware of the domestic violence she was the recipient of. Often times she found herself saying words to victims that she knew she was unable to say to herself, sometimes even with bruises still on her back from the fight the night before, and she would fall further into despair and hopelessness. But she never told anyone, not even her family. It was secret she lived with every day.

The Leap of Faith

The turning point came for her one-day when she was undressing in the locker room. Unbeknownst to her another officer saw the bruises on her back and approached her. She denied it at first; afraid her job was at risk, but when a female sergeant approached her later, offering to help her, she took a chance. This was her first step towards healing the deep pain, isolation and loneliness she felt and thought would never go way. It was also a tremendous leap of faith.

As health care providers and emergency public safety professionals our own needs are often subjugated to the needs of those we serve, both at work and at home.

Creating health (physically, spiritually, emotionally) is a leap of faith. Before we can begin the healing process we must make a paradigm shift, or a systems shift, to a new way of thinking about and being in relationship to, our bodies, our minds, our spirits and our connection with the universe.

Very few people that I know or who have met (including myself) are able to maintain or regain health and wholeness until they make this shift.

Creating health means accepting that there are events in everyone's lives that can not be explained or changed, and at the same time realizing that each of us has conscious input into our state of health and happiness through choosing relationships, thoughts, foods, and activities that support and nourish us fully and completely.

Creating health is also based on the following eternal truth:

Acknowledging, feeling and then releasing rage, guilt, loss, anger and grief is the key to all healing.

The following chapter will provide you with ideas, examples, methods and healing possibilities for the mind, body and spirit. They have assisted many women and men in their journeys towards health and happiness.

Meditation and Stress Management

For those of you in emergency public safety learning something like meditation may sound too over-the-top for you. Yes, you're familiar with the basics and you even tried yoga when you were younger and still a student, but life isn't as simple now as it was then. You're a cop now,or working as an EMT or as a 911 dispatcher.

How will meditation help you roll out to a barricaded suspect or dispatch on an AWD?

Stress is an everyday part of your job, and the adrenaline rush that comes with it is something you've learned to live with and even enjoy at times. Besides, when things go sideways you have your own way of dealing with it and that's been good enough for you up until this point. Why spoil the brew?

At this stage in your career there's nothing that could happen that's so bad that getting a little more sleep or hanging out with the buds won't take care of.

Maybe this is true for you and those you know and work with. Learning to manage your stress differently may make no appreciable difference in your life. No one can argue that sleeping more and socializing regularly with a positive support group isn't important. These factors do contribute to a healthier sense of well-being and are well documented in the scientific literature. However, for those of you who are willing to try something new the benefits of incorporating a regular routine of meditation and yoga into your lives can make all the difference in the world.

Although the allopathic, or traditional western medicine community has long been resistant to alternative or complementary medicine (alternative and complementary medicine has begun showing up in the curriculum of a number of the most prominent medical schools in the country and more are adding it to the basic requirements of a general medical education every year), people have been using these methods for thousands and thousands of years. It's only a matter of time before the research and the quantitative analytic methods of the scientific community catch up and provide the data needed to demonstrate the importance of what people have known for centuries: Faith, prayer, meditation, yoga, chanting and other disciplines of similar kind **work**. Incorporating one or all of these methods into a daily practice has the power to transform lives, including your own. The only person stopping you from reaping the health benefits is you. If you can open yourself up to the possibility of what you may not know yet, then read on. You can pull yourself up by your bootstraps later.

Meditation

Meditation is a lot like martial arts. Once the art is mastered, you'll soon notice that your mind is making a mental assault on the stressors of your life and with minimal effort, you'll learn to step out of the way by returning to whatever the object of your concentration is. Little by little you learn to build up the mental muscles of awareness and then move slowly towards letting go. This is a slow, gentle process. Just as a two year old wanders off and you bring him or her back with gentleness and patience, so it is with the mind. You must bring the same care and gentleness you would bring to that two year old to yourself, without judgment or harshness.

Emergency Public Safety

As someone in emergency public safety approaching yourself with the same kindness and gentleness you may approach a small child may be hard for you to do. Your day-to-day professional life isn't about being soft and gentle. It is often about being direct; taking control of volatile situations, and passing quick judgment over people you've never met before, at least not until you walked in through the front door. Sometimes, despite your best efforts, you are forced to respond with aggression and harshness.

At the end of the day you "put it all away" and go home. Sometimes this easier said then done.

Public Hero, Private Heartache

Typically, in public you are the first to care and respond to the needs of others, and yet in private, the last to care and respond to the needs of yourself, particularly if they are emotional.

If you are working at a large public safety organization you may have access to services that can help you through whatever stressful times you may experience. At the very minimum you can access your own private health insurance and a list of health care providers willing to help you.

If, instead, you are on staff with a small agency in a rural town your access to services provided by someone who doesn't already know you and your entire family may be very limited.

Think of meditation as a tool. You can add it to your tool bag in the same way you might pick up a new jig saw or wrench and not think about it again until you have a need for it, or you can incorporate it into your life and allow it to become a part of who you are everyday, whether you are at work or at home. In this you hold within yourself the power to begin a transformative experience. What does this mean? It means choosing to be aware of what is going on in your body, in your feelings, in your mind, and in the world every day and in every moment of your life.

The Process and The Approach

Most police officers and public safety professionals I know have very high expectations of themselves. Although not all public safety professions require a formal education, most if not all require academy training followed by a probationary period. During this time they are asked to learn new skills and to perform above their own expectations. Their personal limits will be tested and they will be asked and expected to set a new bar for personal and professional performance.

It is also at this time that instructors will impress upon their new recruits and trainees the seriousness and gravity of their newly chosen career field. If there is an underlying unspoken theme here, particularly in the age of litigation and public proliferation of information, it is "thou shalt not make a mistake."

The pressure to conform to this standard is intense and the public and private scrutiny by others constant. Consequently, to succeed many will internalize a compulsive, aggressive, perfectionistic construct that will stay with them long after the probationary period is over, and the career has begun.

This way of viewing the world, and themselves in it will be reinforced on a daily basis by their peers and supervisors as well as by their contact with the public. **Success seems to lie in the hands of those who maintain this public and private persona.**

"You're either for us, or against us."

Blurring the boundary between yourself as a person and yourself as a professional is not uncommon. It is a functional defense as much as it is also nearly an impossible feat to accomplish; that of keeping these two worlds separate. You may want to argue this point, but like it or not our professional lives impact our personal lives, and vice versa, every day we are alive.

If you've ever responded to a child abuse call and then gone home at the end of watch and hugged your own son or daughter a little bit tighter, your personal and professional selves have just intersected.

How can we not blur the boundaries at times? It's a human frailty as well as a human strength. We are above all else human and whether we ask for this or not the people and experiences do touch us .

Few people have the luxury of time to spend in endless hours of deep meaningful contemplation on the mountaintop sorting out the confusion from the chaos, and even if we could find time to contemplate I doubt we could find a space these days that a cell phone couldn't penetrate. Even the Dalai Lama often says he doesn't have time for quiet meditation and reflection. Yet, he has found peace. How can we do the same? How can we transform ourselves?

Today it seems that we have little choice but to assimilate all we experience into our spiritual lives; it is all grist for the mill. The sacred and the mundane are inseparable. Your life is your path. Your disappointments are part of your path; your joys are your path; your last arrest as well as your last arrestee is on your path; ditto your house payments and your last performance evaluation. It's not helpful to wait until you have more time for meditation or contemplation because it may never happen.

Cultivating spirituality, awareness and stress management has to become a full time vocation, and for most of us this has to take place in context of our secular lives here now; in the division; at the station; in the field; on a run and in the air. This is it.

For you, what matters is how you attend to the present moment. This includes motivation, intention, aspiration, desire, hope and expectation. This is not just about what you do, but how you do it. The present moment is where the pedal meets the metal. Your ride on this road depends on how you apply your heart and soul.

What really works then? Is it simply a matter of learning a few new phrases, changing your clothes or hairstyle and breathing deeply? Or do you have to go to the Himalayas, learn to chant, find a guru and learn yoga to transform oneself? I don't think so. To use an old adage all over again: You don't need to see different things, but rather to see things differently.

Meditation As A Power Tool

Approaching meditation in the same way as you've approached other experiences in your life may set you up to fail. Learning to meditate isn't about control or competition. Nor is it about being an expert or doing it better then someone else. It's simply about being mindfully present. That's it.

In fact, learning to be mindfully present is more then enough to begin with, but because your early meditations may consist of your mind wandering or falling asleep, again, you may feel angry and frustrated with yourself. How could something so "simple" be so hard?

If you're like many people who are used to being in control, and knowing how to do things, you may become very judgmental and self-punitive with yourself. This dis-ease may also generate a vague uncomfortable sense of personal inadequacy that you'll be tempted to compartmentalize into the section labeled 'one more frustrating drain on your already limited resources.'

Some of us also harbor feelings of guilt and shame for letting go of other beliefs and practices that were at one time deeply engrained within your character and way of living in the world; beliefs that you were taught and raised with since you were a small child, such as prayer, the presence of God, faith and the need for a spiritual belief in your life, but you have since given up practicing since you became a cop, or EMT, or 911 dispatcher.

It's not that you don't still identify yourself as Baptist or Catholic, or whatever the faith you may have been raised in, but after everything you've seen and witnessed in your career having faith in anything, even the familiar, is a challenge. You know first hand the terrible things people can do in this world, and to each other. How can you can you find the time to meditate when you can't even find the time, or the heart, to practice the beliefs that are familiar to you?

Don't give up.

The images, smells and sounds that leak into your mind during a mediation are compelling ones, particularly if they are emotionally laden. How many people wouldn't have strong feelings about some of the things you've seen? That you would have difficulty refocusing your attention and quieting your mind at times sounds normal given the parameters of your experiences. **Remember this**: a meditation during which there are many thoughts and many attempts to bring the mind back to focus is not a failure, but in fact it is a great training session.

Physiology

Everyone is wired differently from a physiological perspective and each of us brings with us different beliefs and experiences. Therefore, an excellent practice for one person may not at all suit another person. That is OK. Learning what "fits" for you is part of the process. Some people prefer a moving form of mediation such as mindful walking, qi gong, hatha yoga or stretching exercises. Others prefer closed eyes sitting exercises such as concentration, mindfulness meditation, centering prayer or other forms of imaginal centering.

28 DAYS

It really doesn't matter what form you pick, as long as you pick something that feels right for you. Whatever form you feel drawn to practice, make a commitment to practicing it for a full twenty-eight days. Put it into your schedule every day at the same time and do it. This is the basis for forming a healthy habit.

Most people find that waking up fifteen or twenty minutes earlier and doing the practice first thing in the morning not only works well in terms of getting it done, but also sets the tone for a more peaceful, energized, loving and productive day.

More importantly, set aside an increment of time that you can actually do every day, no matter how small (for example: 10 minutes).

If you find yourself able to meditate for more than ten minutes, great, but if not then only do what you have committed to no matter how silly and insignificant it may seem to you at the time. **Build on success.** Don't commit to more than you can actually accomplish.

Setting your target goal too high in the beginning, ("I'll meditate for an hour everyday."), can set you up to fail if you're unable to reach it. You will then add guilt and shame onto a plate that was already too full to begin with and be less inclined to try again.

Remember these key words: **Build On Success**. If ten minutes a day is all you can successfully manage initially, that's ok. Ten minutes it is. What is more important than the actual increment of time is the development of a sustained habit of doing anything for yourself that's not related to work, or family, or whatever else occupies your time and takes you away from caring for yourself.

911

In the world of emergency public safety that can be almost anything, including the suicide you responded to at the end of Watch, or the internal complaints you have yet to finish processing, or the news story that just broke about the homicide you were the sergeant in charge of, or maybe even the birthday party for your kid that you managed to miss yet again because of a body you had to book.

The practice of meditation is one in which eventually all of those feelings and thoughts that are left undone are left behind for discreet periods of time without the aide of unhealthy defenses (overeating, denial, alcohol abuse, rage-attacks, spending sprees, etc.), but until that moment you must at least start with something you can actually accomplish. If ten minutes is the most you can manage and still stay in the room without self-destructing, then ten minutes it is. Gradually, once the habit is established you can increase it to 20 or 30 minutes or whatever increment you are comfortable with.

Remember: Build On Success

Physiological research shows that at least three 20-minute periods of meditation weekly are necessary to experience long term reduction in heart rate, blood pressure, anxiety and other stress related problems.

The following represents a list of some of the more popular methods of meditation. As you review them, keep in mind that not every method works for every person. Some people prefer sitting meditations and can do so for hours on end, while others need a more active form of meditation that works in conjunction with a form of yoga.

Regardless of the method, find one that you are comfortable with and practice it. In the end, once the practice is mastered, to paraphrase the Vietnamese monk Thich Nhat Hanh, one of the most revered Buddhist teachers in the world, every act in life becomes a meditation when done mindfully and fully present.

Breathing Is Life

Learning to breathe is essential to life. This may seem self-evident, but the truth of the matter is it's not. Most of us don't even realize that we've stopped breathing, or that our breathing has changed (becomes more constricted, shallow, rapid) when we're emotionally or physically stressed. We stop breathing so that we can concentrate on the problem at hand.

This is not a conscious act, "I think I'll stop breathing now so I can shoot this suspect." All this happens autonomically, or automatically by our respiratory system as we struggle to regain our focus in a situation that is potentially overwhelming emotionally. So, while we think we know what is happening around us and are responding accordingly, our behaviors and thinking may actually be more affected by our physiological response to stress then we realize. As we begin to hyperventilate, our brain soon experiences the effects of oxygen deprivation. Our thinking may become confused, and our behavior more erratic and reactive. But, if we maintain our calm, deep breathing despite stressful circumstances, we remain relaxed and focused; our body is evenly responsive.

For those of you in law enforcement, think back to when you first learned to shoot. Breathing was tantamount to shooting control and accuracy. Erratic breathing most times led to poor control and missed targets. Learning to breathe through the shots, or controlling the breath, allowed one to maintain focus and take the shot. Likewise, when talking to a hysterical victim, or an injured officer down. The fastest way to maintaining your focus and controlling the scene is through the use of your voice and your breathing. When you feel calm and in control, they feel calmer and more in control, but if you start to hyperventilate, change pitch and fragment, the victim or injured officer soon begins to respond in kind to you. They may panic and behave reactively, placing themselves and others in harms way.

To borrow a line from the movie, Karate Kid, "Wax on, wax off." **Breath equals life.** Learning to use it to your advantage has far reaching effects. Breathing through the events in your life allows you the room to respond, rather then simply react. Meditation is a key that can open this door.

Whatever you learn through alternative methods and disciplines such as meditation, you can take to the street, to the boards and to the rest of your life.

Diaphragmatic and Dantien Breathing

Belly (diaphragmatic) breathing is associated with lower heart rate, reduced blood pressure, increased energy and feelings of peacefulness, relaxation and clarity.

Put one hand on your abdomen and close your eyes. Take a deep breath in through your nose and expel it slowly and completely through your mouth. You will feel your belly flatten. Let the next breath (and all subsequent breaths) come in through your nose. Can you feel your abdomen expand? If you can't, just imagine that a balloon is inflating in your belly when you breathe in and deflating when you breathe out. The out breath is longer than the in breath, like a gentle sigh of relief.

A variant of this technique from Chinese medicine is called Dantien breathing. Dantien means *the field where the elixir of long life is planted.* There are three Dantien, which can be compared to storage batteries for qi, or life-force energy. The largest Dantien is in the lower abdomen. As you breathe, as in belly breathing, you will also notice that your lower back and sides are also expanding and contracting with the breath.

For a fast minibreak any time during the day, take a deep breath in and release it slowly- a letting go breath. Try breathing back from ten to one, one number on each out breath. By the time you get to one, you will notice that your breath is much slower and more regular and that your body mind system is relaxing. With a little practice, you will form the habit of breathing from your diaphragm most of the time.

Concentration Meditation

Concentration meditation is what Herbert Benson, M.D., Harvard cardiologist, first called the Relaxation Response. All forms of meditation in which the mind becomes quiet and focused elicit this innate physiological response, which is the opposite of the body's stress or fight or flight response. Breathing is an important cornerstone of the relaxation response.

Benson first researched the clinically standardized "relaxation" method of meditation in which the word "one" is repeated in time to each outgoing breath. Any word will produce the same results. If you decide to try this you may also wish to choose a word or short series of words that hold special meaning to you. Used in the same way, in conjunction with an outgoing breath, will produce the same results.

An ancient Sanskrit mantra, or meditation focus, is Ham Sah. This is supposed to remind the meditator of the sound of the incoming and outgoing breath. Ham as you breath in, Sah as you breathe out. Ham means 'I am'. Sah means the 'Inner Self', or the 'Divine Spark'.

Any short phrase will work as the meditation focus, either secular or religious. Using phrases such as saying Hail Mary on the in breath, and Full of Grace on the out breath will work equally well and is an excellent focus for those used to repeating the rosary, which is also a kind of concentration meditation. Jewish Meditation by

Rabbi Ari Kaplan, is an excellent primer for Jews. Bensons classic book, The Relaxation Response provides a fine review of secular and religious meditation traditions and practices.

Sitting with your eyes closed, focus on belly or Dantien breathing. Repeat your focus phrase, prayer or mantra in time to either the out breath, or both the incoming or out coming breath if it is a longer phrase. When thoughts come, gently, passively disregard them and return to the repetition. Return to your breath.

Mindful Walking

Thich Nhat Hanh, a Buddhist peace worker, poet and monk, is known for his practice of mindful walking.

Most of the time we are not present to what we are doing. The mind is constantly thinking ahead and behind itself, conjuring up a million thoughts about yesterday and tomorrow, often times perseverating on the negative and completely forgetting about the moment at hand. The only time we actually have, or have any direct control or influence over, is this moment now. John Lennon couldn't have said it any better: Life is what's happening when we're making other plans.

Mindfulness means **being present to what is**, rather than losing ourselves in thoughts about what was and is no longer or what has yet to happen. Mindfulness is an awakening to life, here and now. It is opening up to a nonjudgmental awareness of the wonder of the present moment. As you walk, it's knowing that you are walking, slowly and mindfully.

As you prepare to walk, slowly and mindfully, repeating the cadence of your steps to diaphragmatic breathing or to Hail Marys or whatever you choose. Try repeating a poem such as this one from Being Peace, by Thich Nhat Hanh:

Breathing in I calm body and mind (in breath).
Breathing out I smile (out breath).
Dwelling in the present moment (in breath).
I know this is a wonderful moment (long out breath).

Become aware of the rhythm of your body and breathing. How many steps to your in breath? How many steps to your out breath? How does it feel to move forward, shift your weight, move your feet?

Keeping your breath and body awareness, begin to notice the world around you. See the trees, the grasses, the flowers in season, and the sky. Smell the smells. Hear the sounds. Try to be aware without judgment or reflection. No good or bad sounds. Just sounds.

Nonjudgmental awareness opens the eye of the heart. When you catch yourself thinking about something- and therefore becoming mindless- gently, kindly refocus your attention on breath and body. Do not punish yourself. Recite the poem again and once more become mindful of the world around you.

Easier said then done

This may be challenging for some of you. Mindful Walking is about opening up to what is around you without judgment or reflection, and feeling, as opposed to closing down defensively to what you think you see or feel is around you, or inside of you.

For those of you who are more accustomed to responding to a crime scene, cracking open the chest of a MVA fatal, or calming a PR in the middle of a Domestic Dispute, or who insist on sitting with your back to the wall when having lunch with the kids at a public restaurant, your fanny pack within easy reach, turning off the beacon of hyper vigilance may seem impossible.

Your choice of profession has more or less trained you to be ever vigilant in response to an ever-changing emergent level of need and circumstance. You have learned to process an almost constant stream of information about your environment until it is occurs within you automatically with virtually seamless acuity.

Good portions of the time you're not even aware of your own process because it's been internalized so thoroughly. It is who you are, and you've learned to feel good about this process, or at least safe.

You are also rewarded for your vigilance by your peers, who have also learned to do the same thing with equal accord. You have also learned to delay your feelings and to quickly judge and categorize whatever you see in your environment. Again with the goal of providing the most appropriate immediate response, should a response be needed.

For someone like yourself mindful walking is a leap of faith. You must be willing to suspend the defenses that have become so much a part of who you are every day before you can achieve the benefits of this meditation. Choose your environment very carefully. It must be one that you feel with certainty is safe. If any part of you is remaining hyper vigilant, in preparation for response to a threat, internal or external, real or imagined, this will not work. You may need to start indoors, before going outside into nature, and only then if you can comfortably walk without a need for a hyper vigilant defense. **Build on success**. This isn't a fitness exercise. Its not a competition. This is about letting go and being present to what is.

Sitting Mindfulness Meditation

Sit in your seat with great dignity, back straight and eyes closed. Become aware of your breathing. Notice how the breath is coming in and fills your belly and how breath moves out into space. Feel the coolness of the air on your skin. Keep about 25% of your attention on breathing and the other 75% on the feelings of spacious mindfulness. You may become aware of sounds, sensations and thoughts. Just let them all come and go. Be gentle with yourself. Let them pass across the spacious sky of your mind like clouds. Sogyal Rinpoche, a Tibetan Buddhist Lama, compares the thoughts that arise in mediation to waves that rise from the ocean. It is the ocean's nature to rise. We cannot stop it, but as Rinpoche says, "we can leave the risings in the risings."

Holy Moment Meditation

The concepts of healing and what is holy have a common root in the old Anglo Saxon word haelen, to make whole. Holiness and healing are found in relationship- in our ability to be present in other people, the natural world, the Divine and ourselves.

We have all had holy moments, natural experiences of mindfulness, when our heart opened and we were fully present to a sunrise, a sunset, the sun glinting off a snow covered mountain, lights dancing in the water of a river, the trust felt in holding a new born child to our chest or the look in the eye of someone we love dearly. These are moments of deep and profound gratitude and connection to life, and often we cry when our full heart overflows.

Sit quietly and close your eyes. Focus on belly breathing for a few minutes. Now recall a holy moment and involve all your senses. What did you see? What were the shapes and colors all around you? Can you recall any physical sensations in your body? Any fragrances that come back to you? Any sounds? Were you warm or were you cold? Touching, moving, still? What were you feeling? Where do you experience these emotions in your body? Let the memory fade and return to belly breathing, keeping the focus on the feelings that remain, watching them mindfully, flowing with them. This is the physical sensation of healing and holiness.

Centering Prayer

This form of silent, meditative prayer has been popularized by Father Thomas Keating of Snowmass Monastery in Colorado. You can read about it in his book, Open Mind, Open Heart. The intention of the prayer is to be in God's presence. The idea is to shift awareness away from the thoughts that Keating compared to "boats floating down the river of consciousness to the river itself." The river is God's presence, that loving life force in which we live and move and have our own being.

Prior to beginning the practice, choose a prayer word, a Sacred Word, which will serve as your reminder to let go of the thoughts and re-enter the river of the Divine Presence. The prayer word can be anything that reminds you of your intention to keep your appointment with God. Peace, Shalom, Hail Mary, Great Spirit, Goddess Energy, The Lord is My Shepherd, are a few examples. Before you start even your first session, center yourself any way you choose and pray for a scared word to come to you. Once you have chosen one, keep it for at least a month. Changing it in the midst of prayer is a distraction.

Center yourself in the silent intention to be present to God. There is no focus on the breath at all in this practice. When you notice your mind wandering, repeat the Sacred Word a few times until you can let go once again as gently as laying a feather on a piece of cotton.

As with all forms of meditation, don't worry about how well you are doing. As Keating writes, "the feeling that we are in God's Presence is a kind of grace. The best any of us can do is to have a willing heart by intentionally entering silence and waiting there for the Divine Beloved."

The Egg of Light Healing Exercise

One of the most ancient forms of healing and concentration consists of imagining yourself in the center of an egg of Divine Light. Sit quietly with eyes closed and imagine a great star of loving light above you. Feel streams of light washing over you and invite it to enter the top of your head and wash down through your body like a river washes through the sand on its bottom, carrying away fatigue, fear, dis-ease or negativity. As all the darkness washes out of the bottoms of your feet imagine that it is taken in by Mother Earth and turned to compost. Spend a little extra time washing any part of your body where there is tension, pain or disease.

Let the light wash clean the boundaries of your heart, revealing the inner light, which is your own true essence. Let that heart light shine more and more brightly, filling your cells and tissues and extending beyond your body---three feet above and below you and on all sides until you feel as though you are sitting in an egg of healing, protective light. Affirm that all positive thoughts and prayers from others will penetrate the egg and reach you, but all negative influences will bounce back off the egg and a blessing be returned to their sender. Affirm that all your own positive thoughts will reach through to others, and all negative thoughts will bounce back off the inner shell of the egg and a blessing of compassion will return to awaken you heart to love.

Loving Kindness Meditation

Meditate any way that you choose for a few minutes, or enter the egg of light. Then repeat those blessings first for yourself, then for your loved ones, then for those you are in conflict with, and then for the world. I like to imagine the star of light from the prior exercise expanding into a circle of light into which I call those to be blessed by name, imagining them as fully as possible.

Here are the blessings:

May I be at peace. May my heart remain open. May I awaken to the light of my own true nature. May I be healed. May I be a source of healing for all beings.

See a circle of Divine Light. Invite your loved ones into it, calling them by name. See them in as much detail as you possible.

Imagine the loving light shining down on them and washing through them, revealing the light within their own hearts. Then bless them:

May you be at peace. May your heart remain open. May you awaken to the light of your own true nature. May you be healed. May you be a source of healing for all beings.

Next, think of those people who you hold in judgment, and to whom you are ready to begin extending forgiveness. Place them in a circle of light and see the light washing away all their negativity, just as it did for you and your loved ones. Bless them:

May you be at peace. May your heart remain open. May you awaken to the light of your own true nature. May you be healed. May you be a source of healing for all beings.

See our beautiful planet as it appears from outer space, a delicate jewel suspended in the vastness of infinite space. Imagine the Earth surrounded by light, the green continents, the blue waters, the white polar caps. The two leggeds and the four leggeds, the fish that swim, the birds that fly, those that creep and crawl on the brown earth. Earth is a place of opposites. Day and night, good and evil, up and down, male and female. Be spacious enough to hold it all as you offer these blessings:

May there be peace on Earth. May the hearts of all people be open to themselves and to each

other. May all people awaken to the light of their own true nature. May all creation be blessed and be a blessing to All That Is.

Bone Marrow Cleansing Exercise from Qi gong

The entire bone marrow cleansing exercise, plus many other excellent exercises are on Ken Cohen's award winning video tape, The Way of Qi gong, Sounds True, PO Box 8010, Boulder, CO, 80306. In brief, there are four steps:

Step One: Cup hands and lift arms as though carrying a small ball, bring hands into prayer pose. Think of the entire universe being present within your heart. Hold this standing mediation for about a minute. Let arms drift down to your sides.

Step Two: Palms forward, raise arms to or about shoulder level, and then turn palms away from body. Think of yourself as filling the universe. Hold for about a minute. Let arms drift downwards till they rest by your sides.

Step three: This is the only repetitive step, (two to five times each side). Tuck the back of one hand against the lower spine. Raise the other hand, palm forward to the sky. Gather the qi from all the sources that are meaningful to you (I call this "waving to the universe"). Energetically connect the palm of your hand to the crown of the head (Don't actually touch the top of your head) and draw down the qi, moving your hand parallel to and in front of your body. Imagine that you are drawing the qi down through the marrow of your bones, visualizing your skeleton. Imagine that any old qi as darkness being pushed out through the feet into the mother earth for recycling. When the hand that is bringing the qi down reaches the level of the hand against your lower back, change hands and repeat on the other side.

Cup the hands up and raise them as if lifting a large beach ball. When the hands are above the head turn them palms up and stand for a moment like a tree connecting earth to heaven. Gather the qi, make an energetic connection of both hands to the crown, and then draw down the qi through the bones with both hands.

Appendix 1

The Angry Dispatcher: Fact or Fiction

.

I've lost track of how many times I've been told by someone that dispatchers are just a particular breed of person and that's why the dispatch floor's a rough place to be. "It's a snake pit out there. It's too bad it's gotta be like that, but that's the way it's always been. That's the way it will always be. This job will change you and if you don't toughen up you'll just be eaten alive."

You know, I've always believed there's a little bit of truth in everything, but from my experience life doesn't necessarily have to be about "eat or be eaten." Sometimes there comes a point when you have to draw the line and make a choice.

I don't think anyone will argue with me that dispatchers have to possess certain skills and to some extent certain personality characteristics that will enable he or she to do the job. Not everyone can do this job, or do it well.

We know all the obvious qualities that a dispatcher needs to succeed: multitasking, typing speed, ability to make accurate decisions quickly and while under pressure, etc. etc, but we often leave out some of the most critical elements to dispatching. Dispatchers must also learn to develop an internal mechanism or defense that will allow them to tolerate extreme levels of pressure, stress and verbal abuse, routinely experienced, all while performing their jobs to within acceptable standards. Few, however, are willing to admit or acknowledge at what cost this success comes to them. Even fewer are recognized for this daily sacrifice of the self.

"Well, after a while it all becomes routine. It's no big deal. You take one suicide call, you take a hundred suicide calls."

Routines are mechanisms we develop to help us cope with our lives. They keep us organized and allow us to remain on task during more mundane activities. When applied to public safety, where any one dispatcher can take literally hundreds of calls daily that fall far outside the range of "normal" behavior and experience for most people, the threshold by which we define mundane radically changes.

In short, we are now referring to the consistent ability to create structure where there may be none, and the ability to remain organized and functional during crisis and extraordinary levels of stress.

This is a fundamental skill for any type of emergency public safety work. Well-rehearsed routines and training are the core elements that enable one to respond to crisis situations. Yet, despite this truism and the ability to get the job done, responding to certain types of calls, (i.e.:

suicide, officer down, child death), on an emotional and psychological level, are never routine.

Dispatchers routinely dispatch on calls from polite appropriate John or Jane Q. Public dutifully calling in to report a cat up a tree. But by and large, the majority of calls are not from John and Jane Q. Public. They are from individuals who are calling because they are in crisis, and whether their crisis is real or imagined, at the time they call they feel their crisis is real. They are not particularly concerned with how dispatchers feel when they take the call nor are they worried about how inappropriate or unreasonable they may be during the call, while they are talking to you, the dispatcher.

Dispatchers may spend hours on calls from angry, out-of-control, verbally abusive, sometimes 5150 individuals who insist that their failure to take charge of their lives constitutes an emergency on your part, but that's the job. It comes with the territory.

Just like my job, no one ever comes to see me because they're happy and then when they start feeling better, they leave; it comes with the territory. Sometimes they don't even say good-bye. Do I have feelings about it? Sure, but why fight it? If I plan to do the job then I have to accept that this, too, is part of what I will experience every day I decide to show up to work.

Throughout my work I continue to be impressed with the incredible professionalism of dispatchers. Quite honestly, I don't think I could do the job. As a psychologist, I admit to my limitations. I can only listen to one person at a time. I am happy to leave multitasking to the professionals.

The dispatchers I meet and work with do a fantastic job of handling an incredibly broad range of critical situations, while still managing to have personal lives, take care of families, do volunteer work and take on additional tasks and duties. It boggles the mind sometimes when I realize the sheer volume, range in magnitude and intensity of calls experienced by a dispatcher during a single day and yet still managing to maintain a professional decorum and a sense of humor.

On the other hand I've also seen this job take its toll on human lives, as good kind decent people become angry, bitter and resentful. Lives are changed, and sometimes there appears no turning back.

The destructive effects of anger are well documented. Anger is the single most significant cause of disease and premature death in individuals. In studies completed by Redford Williams (Duke University) and Robert Sapolsky (Standford University) anger, rage and hostility were shown to be particularly damaging to the cardiovascular system. Anger is a major risk in heart disease and at least equal to or perhaps greater than the traditionally recognized risk factors such as high cholesterol and high blood pressure.

As a psychologist and a consultant I've been in a position to listen to many things and I've heard many explanations for this behavioral change. One of the most popular has been one offered by supervisors and command staff, and sometimes even dispatchers themselves, who say that dispatchers are simply an aggressive, hostile group of people who are this way by nature, whether they are at home or at work. They are born that way; I've heard people say, as though somewhere on their DNA there's a genetic marker for "angry dispatcher".

You and I both know that there is always the exception to the rule. There will always be a small percentage of people who, no matter where you put them, are angry, hostile individuals and they don't care who knows it, but even these people did not start out that way. Unless you're a sociopath everyone was once "someone's baby boy or girl," even dispatchers.

For years now, I've been asking dispatchers what their hopes, dreams and expectations were when they first came on the job, and you know what I found out? **Not one** has ever said, "When I came on the job I wanted to forget how to feel. I wanted to become angry and hostile to everyone around me, including my family," nor did anyone ever say "When I came on the job I wanted to be abused for hours all day long, and then if I complain, or cry, or feel sad because someone dies on my watch I want to be humiliated by my co-workers for being weak and "unable to take it."

In fact, just the opposite is true. 98 per cent of the dispatchers I talk to say that when they first came on the job they wanted to make a difference; to help people; to do something they could feel proud of; to provide a stable income for their homes and family; to be challenged and stimulated by the work they do and to feel respected and listened to by their supervisors and colleagues. Is this so unreasonable or surprising? No, these are basic human needs and beliefs, and feelings we all can relate to and perhaps even want for ourselves.

So what happens? How does someone go from being an idealistic, hopeful new employee who believes in good things happening to good people to being seen as angry, mean and hostile? Does it happen overnight, or is this a long process? How do you stop it?

First comes the decision to change.

This process that dispatchers are inadvertently placed in the middle of is one that is endemic to the work. Long-term exposure to critical levels of stress leads to burnout and when left untreated ultimately results in behavioral, physical and psychological change. Said another way, dispatching is ripe for burnout and manna from heaven for developing posttraumatic stress disorder, widely undiagnosed amongst dispatchers.

Few people can do the work of dispatching and not care. As with any helping profession, most individuals first starting out are deeply committed to their work. It is at this time, more then any other time in their career, that they willing to go 110%. It is also the time they are the most vulnerable to burnout. Because of the nature of the work, they begin to redefine themselves and soon, as a way of coping with the stress of the job, their sense of self becomes intrinsically wrapped up into the work that they do. Their identity is now no longer separated from their profession. By and large, excluding individual variability, in time they become one in the same. As long as things go well and according to expectations, the individual belief system is intact, but when and if this is not the case serious problems can develop.

Research on stress and burnout suggests that when ones hopes, dreams and expectations become frustrated; they become our greatest source of stress and burnout. Once active, resourceful, energetic workers become disillusioned resentful and angry.

Dispatchers are no different then other helping professionals. Committed to the job, they care greatly and when something goes sideways, they feel it deeply. In the same way that taking the job to begin with is a leap of faith, so is doing the work day after day. You must have faith that the work you do really does make a difference; that the sacrifice of yourself is worthwhile in the long run and that the stress and abuse you are willing to tolerate is worth it. You do so because you believe that through your work you are contributing to something greater than yourself and, despite how difficult it can be for reasons that are never expected, you stay in because it means something to you about who you are. Like the existential quest for meaning, every day you spend as a dispatcher is a day spent contributing to something greater than us all.

But dispatching is not a profession that reaps rewards and public recognition. In fact, most dispatchers rarely find out about the outcome of a call let alone receive positive feedback from peers, supervisors or the agencies they work for. Their best work often goes unnoticed, but whenever a mistake is made or complaint is taken, the agencies are first to notice. This, in combination with the daily exposure to trauma and extreme levels of stress, without treatment, recognition or intervention, and I say we have found the source of most dispatcher's anger, or shall I say rage.

Like everything in life, transformation is a process. I know I'm not telling you a news flash. For many years dispatching wasn't even seen as a profession. Dispatchers were "those people who answered the telephone" and so, consequently those on the outside believed there was nothing to the job. How could there a problem if all you do is answer the telephone? What's the big deal? Why should you have feelings about anything? You're not out in the field. You don't have any right to have feelings. The people outside, they have the right to have feelings.

Even dispatchers who may have felt differently when they first began their careers, after a few years on the boards would agree. They had stopped feeling very much of anything at work, except for one feeling: anger. Anger they could get a hold of in a heartbeat, no problem, ask anyone and they'll tell you. To be a good dispatcher you have to have attitude, or you won't make it, but this is wrong thinking. **It's time to set the record straight.**

You have the right to have feelings, and to feel angry, sad, depressed, or even want to cry because someone you've been on the line with for three hours has just taken his or her own life. This does not mean that you are weak, or flawed. It does mean that you are human, and being human is a good thing. It is a very good thing.

I once spoke to group of dispatchers in Sacramento and as we talked about feelings, one of them said, "If I start to feel things now, I don't know if I can stop! So, I'm not even going to go there."

OK, but if you don't go there now, then when? What has to happen to get your attention? Do you have to develop high blood pressure? or get stopped for a DUI? or wait until your marriage breaks up because you've lost your temper one too many times, again? or maybe you should have an affair? That ought to clear things up.

When I see or hear about an angry dispatcher with attitude, I see someone who is burned out. I see someone who probably started out full of hopes and dreams and expectations and then became frustrated, disappointed or disillusioned by the job, by the experience, by the organization or maybe even by how little they actually have control over. I see someone who continues to come to the table and does their job yet loses a little bit more of themselves every day, and who, whether they like it or notice it or not, takes the job home with them day after day. I see someone whose anger is really about feeling helpless and hopeless to change what's happening around them, and what's happening to them.

This is a tough job and it will change you and for some things there's nothing you can do about it. Being a psychologist has changed some aspects of who I am, and that's the nature of the beast, I accept that but I also choose to go there. I also choose to keep what is important to me, about who I am and about my life. It is always a choice, and in accepting that then you must also know that you deserve to be here.

You have the right to happiness. You have the right to be treated with respect, and human dignity. You have the right to your feelings no matter what they are, whether someone agrees or disagrees with you. The dispatch center as a "pit of snakes" filled with "angry hostile" dispatchers "waiting to devour you alive" only has to be that way if you decide to keep it that way. What's your choice?

NORTH SHORE PUBLISHING AND EDUCATIONAL SERVICES
dr911.com™

Quick Order Form

☎ **Telephone orders:** Call 213-864-7661. Have your credit card ready.

💻 **email orders:** orders@dr911.com

✉ **Postal orders:** North Shoe Publishing and Educational Services, P.O. Box 9865, Las Vegas, NV 89191. USA. Telephone: 213-864-7661

Please send the following books, discs or reports. I understand that I may return any of them for a full refund- for any reason, no questions asked.

____

____

____

Please send more FREE information on:
Other books Speaking/seminars Mailing lists Consulting

Name: ________________________________
Address: ________________________________
City: ________________ State _____ Zip ________

Telephone: ________________
Email address: ________________________

Sales tax: Please add 7.75% for products shipped to California addresses.

Shipping by air:
US: $4 for the first book or disc and $2.oo for each additional product.
International: $9 for the first book or disc; $5 for each additional product (estimate).

Payment: Cheque Credit Card
Visa Mastercard Optima AMEX Discover

Card number: ____________________________
Name on card: ___________________________
Exp. Date: _____________________________

NORTH SHORE PUBLISHING AND EDUCATIONAL SERVICES
dr911.com™

Quick Order Form

☎ **Telephone orders:** Call 213-864-7661. Have your credit card ready.

💻 **email orders:** orders@dr911.com

✉ **Postal orders:** North Shoe Publishing and Educational Services, P.O. Box 9865, Las Vegas, NV 89191. USA. Telephone: 213-864-7661

Please send the following books, discs or reports. I understand that I may return any of them for a full refund- for any reason, no questions asked.

____

____

____

Please send more FREE information on:
Other books Speaking/seminars Mailing lists Consulting

Name: ______________________________
Address: ____________________________
City: ______________ State _____ Zip ________

Telephone: ________________
Email address: ________________________

Sales tax: Please add 7.75% for products shipped to California addresses.

Shipping by air:
US: $4 for the first book or disc and $2.oo for each additional product.
International: $9 for the first book or disc; $5 for each additional product (estimate).

Payment: Cheque Credit Card
Visa Mastercard Optima AMEX Discover

Card number: ____________________________
Name on card: ___________________________
Exp. Date: _____________________________

NORTH SHORE PUBLISHING AND EDUCATIONAL SERVICES

dr911.com™

Quick Order Form

☎ **Telephone orders:** Call 213-864-7661. Have your credit card ready.

💻 **email orders:** orders@dr911.com

✉ **Postal orders:** North Shoe Publishing and Educational Services, P.O. Box 9865, Las Vegas, NV 89191. USA. Telephone: 213-864-7661

Please send the following books, discs or reports. I understand that I may return any of them for a full refund- for any reason, no questions asked.

____

____

____

Please send more FREE information on:
Other books Speaking/seminars Mailing lists Consulting

Name: ________________________________
Address: ________________________________
City: ________________ State ______ Zip ________

Telephone: ____________________
Email address: __________________________

Sales tax: Please add 7.75% for products shipped to California addresses.

Shipping by air:
US: $4 for the first book or disc and $2.oo for each additional product.
International: $9 for the first book or disc; $5 for each additional product (estimate).

Payment: Cheque Credit Card
Visa Mastercard Optima AMEX Discover

Card number:______________________________
Name on card: ____________________________
Exp. Date: ______________________________